D0497727

101 Things To Do Before You DIET

101 Things To Do Before You DIET

MIMI SPENCER

Doubleday

LONDON · TORONTO · SYDNEY · AUCKLAND · JOHANNESBURG

TRANSWORLD PUBLISHERS
61–63 Uxbridge Road, London W5 5SA
A Random House Group Company
www.rbooks.co.uk

First published in Great Britain in 2009 by Doubleday
an imprint of Transworld Publishers

Copyright ©Mimi Spencer 2009

Mimi Spencer has asserted her right under the Copyright,
Designs and Patents Act 1988 to be identified as the author
of this work.

A CIP catalogue record for this book is available from the
British Library.

ISBN 9780385616102

This book is sold subject to the condition that it shall not,
by way of trade or otherwise, be lent, resold, hired out, or
otherwise circulated without the publisher's prior consent
in any form of binding or cover other than that in which it
is published and without a similar condition, including this
condition, being imposed on the subsequent purchaser.

Addresses for Random House Group Ltd companies outside
the UK can be found at: www.randomhouse.co.uk
The Random House Group Ltd Reg. No. 954009

The Random House Group Limited supports The Forest
Stewardship Council (FSC), the leading international forest-
certification organization. All our titles that are printed
on Greenpeace-approved FSC-certified paper carry the
FSC logo. Our paper procurement policy can be found
at www.rbooks.co.uk/environment

Typeset in Bodoni Old-face and Thesis
Designed by Smith & Gilmour, London
Printed and bound in Australia by
Griffin Press

2 4 6 8 10 9 7 5 3 1

For Lily May

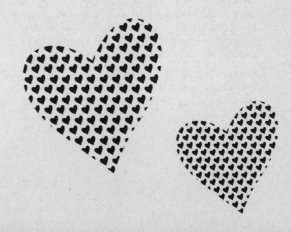

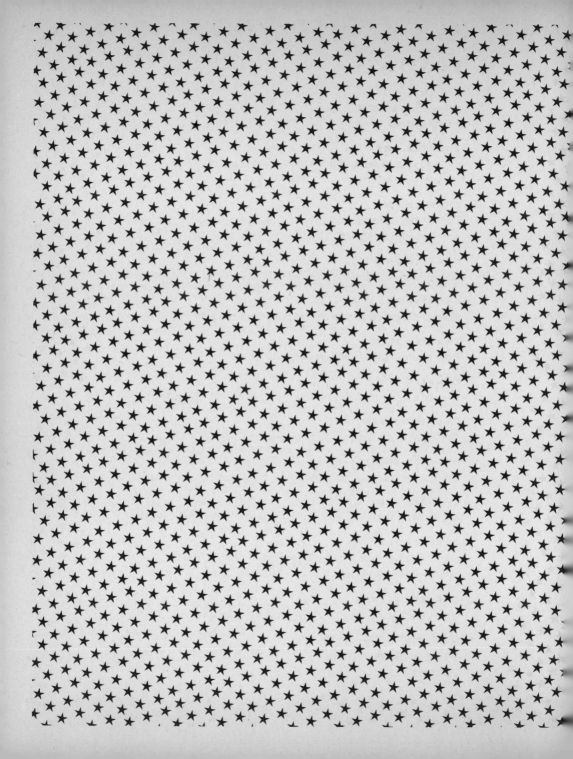

CONTENTS

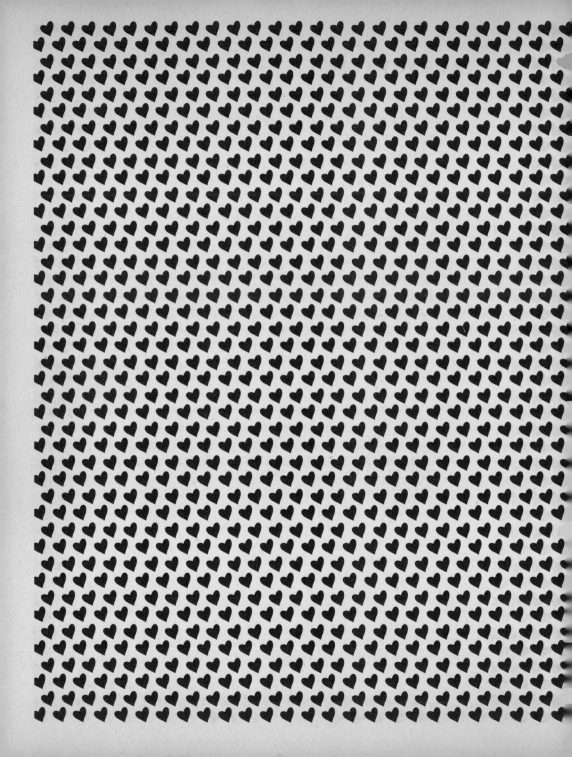

ACKNOWLEDGEMENTS

Thanks and a big iced bun to Lizzy Kremer, a woman of great insight who knows that a dessert with two spoons is still well worth having.

I also owe a triple helping of gratitude to Marianne Velmans, my voice of reason, and to all at Transworld, particularly Manpreet Grewal, Alison Barrow, Kate Samano, Sarah Roscoe and Janine Giovanni.

Special thanks to Nicola Jeal for constant bloody brilliance over more years than I care to count, and to Sue Peart at You Magazine for lending me five years of column space in which to debate the state of the nation's wardrobe.

And finally, always, my thanks to Paul, Lily and Ned, the loves of my life.

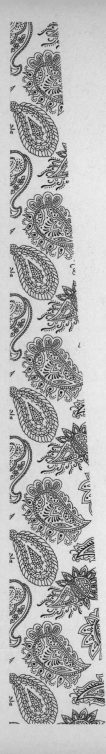

INTRODUCTION
THIN: THE DREAM OF A GENERATION

I don't know a woman who wouldn't like to lose half a stone. Some, of course, would dearly love to lose more – a dress size or two – but most of us gaze mistily into the middle distance of our lives and envisage a time when we'll be, ooh, seven pounds lighter, a time when a size-12 skirt doesn't pinch after lunch, when our jeans won't clutch at our thighs like a petulant toddler, when our stomach is more buff than muffin. For most of us, it's an irritating, persistent hum in the back-rooms of our mind.

I'm not about to tell you to stop aspiring to be that bit slimmer. As a forty-year-old woman with a healthy interest in looking fabulous in a clingy top, I recognize the desire which burns within all of us to make the very best of what we've got. I'm well aware of the female need to compete with our peers – how we all look at the bikini bodies on the beach to gauge whether we measure up, how bloody brilliant it feels to walk into a crowded room and know that people are sizing up the wiggle in your walk and not the wobble in your chin. Really, who doesn't want to look better, feel happier, be fitter? We want to be in control of our lives. We want our appearance to reflect our aspirations – in our careers, for our children, for our sense of self. In short, and given the choice, most of us don't want to be fat.

This book is the simple, signposted route to achieving that goal. It nails exactly how you can arrive at a whole new you, a place where you'll feel, look and *be* better than you ever have before. The difference is that I know you can do all of this *without dieting* (listen carefully and you can hear little angels singing). So don't expect self-flagellation, self-denial, weigh-ins, wailing and nothing but grapefruit at every meal for the next six weeks. Instead, step by step, in 101 ways, you'll discover:

- ✱ How to stop judging and start living.
- ✱ How to eat more and weigh less.
- ✱ How to dress thin and look gorgeous.
- ✱ How to change your mind to change your shape.
- ✱ How to banish body blues and find body balance.
- ✱ How dieting is the problem, not the solution.

This, then, is a real-time book with a realistic promise: it will examine your relationship with your fork, your fridge, your fashion, your friends, your foibles. It nudges open the secrets of how we really feel about our bodies, and, in particular, those bits we'd rather lock in a box and never meet again. It looks at why we've become a nation of marshmallows, flumped in front of our computer or TV screen, and how we can ease ourselves off the sofa and into a better body, while remaining – gloriously – in the comfort zone. And here's the cherry on the cake: unlike a diet, it delivers effective answers *today* – not tomorrow, not after the weekend, not when Christmas has turned into January. But now.

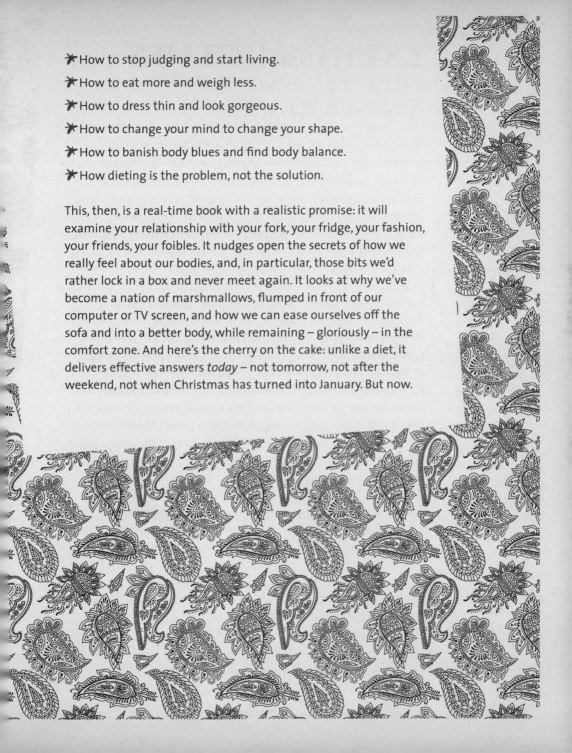

THE FAT OF THE LAND: HOW DIETING CONSUMED US ALL

It's odd, isn't it, that in a world beset by knife crime, credit crisis, impending peak-oil and looming ecological meltdown, we should spend so very much time thinking about how much we weigh? It is, if you like, a metaphor for our times: while Rome, or its equivalent, burns, we're gazing at our navels and wondering who ate all the pies.

Latest figures suggest that it's we Brits who are wolfing down a fair few of them. Britain has now been officially classified as the Fat Man of Europe, although I'm sure I met the actual Fat Man of Europe a few months back on a long-haul trip to Miami. This man leaked over into my space like an oil spill, making it exceedingly difficult for me to concentrate on my glossy magazine, a publication which contained so many skinnifers, so many lovely bones, that it nearly rattled when I took it out of my handbag.

There are many curious aspects to our current obsession with body shape, but perhaps the most alarming is that the more we scrutinize the rack-thin celebrity A-list, the fatter we get. The gulf between the Eats and the Eat-Nots is now wider – literally – than ever. While a growing number of us are expanding at breakneck speed, the rest are panic-dieting, eating only papaya or mackerel or things that begin with G.

For my part, I seem to have been on a diet since the moment my first child arrived – bringing with her a whole heap of joy, but leaving behind a whole lot of disheartening body issues: the heavier hips, the wider thighs, the belly hell-bent on heading south, boobs in close pursuit. Like many women, I have ricocheted between fashionable It Diets. I've tried Atkins, GI, South Beach, Hay, Montignac, Perricone, Caveman, Combining . . . I have done egg-white omelettes, maple-syrup detox, cabbage soup in a Thermos flask, a Dulcalax at bedtime, a Slim-a-Soup for lunch . . . Ring any bells? If there is one activity that really binds British women together, it's our shared obsession with dieting. Four out of ten of us are *permanently on a diet*; it's our national hobby, our favourite sport. A recent survey found that 40 per cent of women had undergone a 'deprivation diet' at least once. Indeed, it's almost hard not to, such is the supply of quick-fix advice out there if you're fool enough to buy it. Though we know it's all useless, a hiding to nothing, we persist. Another fat-blasting super-diet strolls up the path and that's it. Something inside crumbles. A plaintive little voice within bleats, *This might be The One*. There is, after all, something hugely provocative about the possibility of losing weight, the scrap of an idea that you'll shrink. It wins me over every time. And every time, I lose. Not weight, so much as the will to live.

'If there is one activity that really binds British women together, it's our shared obsession with dieting. Four out of ten of us are *permanently on a diet*; it's our national hobby, our favourite sport.'

DIETING? THAT'S NO WAY TO LOSE WEIGHT

It doesn't take a genius to see the deep paradox at the heart of our modern relationship with food: the more obsessed we are about 'healthy' eating, the fatter (and more miserable) we have become. For every 'diet book' that hits the shelves, we put on an extra pound; for every 'make me skinny' TV show, we let out the belt by one more liberating notch.

Clearly, none of it works – not the deprivation, not the faddism, not in the long run. It's worth knowing that the average New Year dieter cracks after seventy-eight days – just, by some cruel twist, in time for Easter. All we know for sure is that dieting leaks the enjoyment out of food. It leaves us lost. And the technicians in the diet-food labs want to keep it that way. Just imagine if they alighted on a dream product which *actually* made us slim and kept us there. They'd be out of a job faster than you can say aspartame.

In fact, conventional diet strategies are believed to have a success rate of just 5 per cent. There's such a wealth of evidence pointing up this cheerless fact that a team of psychologists at UCLA has conducted a comprehensive survey of thirty-one long-term diet studies in order to unleash the inviolable truth. 'Several studies indicate that dieting is actually a consistent predictor of future weight *gain*,' said their analysis, published in *American Psychologist*. 'We asked what evidence there is that dieting works in the long term, and found that the evidence shows the opposite.' They discovered that, although people who go on slimming diets can indeed shed several pounds in the first few months, the vast majority return to their original weight within five years, while at least a third end up heavier than when they embarked on the project. All that will-power. All that punishment. All for nothing. The report concluded that it's better not to diet at all: 'You're no worse off, and you spare your body all the damage associated with having a yo-yoing physique.'

If you want fries with that, a 2003 study found that the more children and teenagers dieted, the more likely they were to become obese adults. Some experts now argue that obesity is increasingly a disease caused by its treatment. It is thought that parents who impose strict diets on their children, or who engage in faddy diets themselves, send the message to their kids that food is dangerous. Something to fear. As a result, many of us are increasingly anxious around food, alarmed by E numbers and E-coli, by pesticides and food miles, by salt and sugar, fat and cholesterol and other anti-nutrient evils waiting to corrupt our innocent forks.

In this climate of dread, it's hardly surprising we're in a spin. For many in this freaky world, food is no longer sustenance and succour, but the work of Beelzebub. This century has also seen the rise of the Extreme Diet – regimes which are harsh, restrictive, proscriptive and (quite possibly) downright dangerous, programmes which urge us to drop a food group to drop a dress size, or to sniff a vanilla bean to annihilate those hunger pangs. Many of us roller-coast from fat fear to thin spin, ever eager for the Next Big Idea (preferably with a celebrity fan-base) which promises to erase the apron belly and the bingo wing, the muffin top and the triple boob, or whatever new term the weekly mags have seized upon to pinpoint another ugly body zone and put it on parade.

YOUR BODY, YOUR PROBLEM: HOW FOOD BECAME THE ENEMY AND FAT BECAME TABOO

Part of the problem is that calories are everywhere, beckoning, beguiling. There's the cheap alcohol, the nightly bottle of Shiraz. The coffee and croissant culture. The explosive portion sizes. We're short of time, so we drive rather than walk. We're short of expertise, so our evenings are punctuated by the ping of the microwave. We eat on the go, we multi-task during meals, picking up something or other and shovelling it in at the traffic lights (consider the dispiriting thought that more Americans eat lunch in the car than in a restaurant). Food is everywhere, and if it's not food profusion, it's food porn, turning our humble daily bread into something to worship which costs eight quid at an artisan deli. No wonder we're overwhelmed.

And all this, don't forget, comes in an era of food fascism, where every mouthful is graded, guided and laced with guilt, an era in which women obsess about their bodies every fifteen minutes (which is, apparently, more than men think about sex). A third of women admit to using slimming pills and laxatives, and 98 per cent of us recently told a magazine survey that we HATE our bodies. Such dysfunction leads to some spectacularly bizarre behaviour. Chew over the fact that in the UK we spend £3 billion a year on fast food, £3.6 billion on chocolate ... and £2 billion on diet products. Isn't that absurd?

The only comforting thing for me about all this is that it's not just my problem. It's yours too. We're all at it. In my travels as a fashion journalist, the women I encounter often seem stricken by a paralysing body crisis, spending their entire life – the only one they'll ever get – feeling bad because they're feeling fat. An unconscionable waste, sure; but I know how real the body blues can be. I've been there too. In fact, I've got the T-shirt (a huge baggy one with DON'T LOOK AT ME! emblazoned on the front in big bold letters). When I gained weight after having children, I too felt dumpy, dreary, about as sassy and engaging as a sideboard. It seemed that my body shape could, with an extra few pounds here or there, dictate the very shape of my day. Like so many women, I spent years attempting to keep up, trying to slim down, poring over calorie charts, gleaning juicy little tips from celebrity trainers and Hollywood chefs, using every ounce of will-power to stop myself succumbing to the pull of the all-butter flapjack or that last, provocative roast potato.

But one day – a good day, a strong day – I'd had enough. I came to my senses. I'm still me, I thought. I'm just wearing slightly bigger trousers. I looked at the research. I looked at my life, trapped between the bedroom mirror and the bathroom scales, eaten up with the dull minutiae of weight control. I realized that not only was serial dieting an appalling waste of time, energy, money, conversation and emotion – it was also, ultimately, utterly pointless. That was the final ignominy of it all: in the long run, dieting doesn't work, won't work, can't work – and will almost certainly leave us worse off. So I stopped. Right there.

As a consequence, I started to write less about John Galliano's organdie kimonos and whether Prada made sense (the jury's out), and more about grittier, bread-and-butter issues: our connection with our bodies, our need to be contenders, how our shape – the shape of the nation – is changing (fast), why we're so very obsessed with dieting – and how, vitally, it just doesn't seem to get us anywhere.

But if dieting was a fraud, then what *would* work? What could serve up the dream of slim without the demands of Hay, Atkins, Zone and the rest? What was needed, it seemed to me, was a *live-it*, not a diet: something practical, sustainable, effective – holistic, even – a way of life that viewed my appetite as part of a wider picture, a realistic picture which encompassed my body image, self-esteem, lifestyle and the regular ups and downs of my normal life, and not one only suitable for Hollywood starlets, heiresses, models and people who have staff to juice their morning beetroot.

As I began to compile this book, it became clear that the missing element in most best-selling diets is confidence. Self-belief. Once you harness this magic ingredient – and this book will reveal how, in bite-sized, transformative helpings – the slim you is a natural progression. In writing this book, I ditched the diets and started to find ways to feel better about being me. And guess what? I lost that pesky half stone.

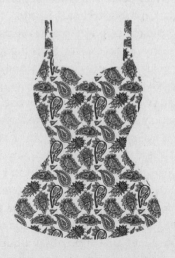

THE 101 PROMISE

Here, then, is the no-diet diet. This book will help you to lose weight – really – but it will also show you how to access your slender self. It is a book of directions, not rules. It's about tips and cheats, small things that collectively will make a big difference. There's a pick 'n' mix quality to it, partly because reading eighty thousand words of dense copy will lead you inexorably to the biscuit tin – but mostly because some of the things detailed within will be your ticket out of here, and some just won't. Here are 101 suggestions to skinny yourself, a veritable smorgasbord of advice, and introducing even half of them into your everyday life (yes, your *everyday life* – this is no two-week, quick-fix regime, but a life-changing, never-going-back, *Thelma and Louise* sort of book) will make all the difference in the world. Some are practical, others psychological. Some are a bit of fun, some are a bit of work. There are new methods and old wisdom. You'll discover a comprehensive examination of the artifice, the subterfuge, the dodges and the dives that are the staples of the fashion insider, tips that will make you seem sensationally slimmer at a stroke.

For every ploy, plot and ruse to slim you down, there's a practical pointer that will make a tangible difference to your shape. There are countless simple strategies for calorie skimming, and an in-depth look at how our weight is ultimately, intimately related to how we feel. You'll learn how to normalize your relationship with food and why bringing it to the forefront of your daily routine, rather than tucking it in between all your other responsibilities, might just obviate the need for serial-dieting, binge-eating, panic-snacking and guilt-tripping. Oh, and it will also get you into smaller jeans.

This book will encourage a common-sense, eminently feasible approach. If you think it's time to free yourself from the billboard babes, from the tyranny of thin, from the curse of being on a constant diet, then this is for you. While we're at it, we will also slaughter the diet myth, the masochism, the self-inflicted misogyny. This book will teach you to down weapons and end the war with your own self-image. The first step is to start to love the skin you're in. Don't compare yourself to friends, models, sisters, celebrities, that girl in your yoga class who always looks so great in lemon-yellow sweatpants. It's a trap, and you could spend your entire life down that particular pit. Be kind to yourself and you're on the first rung out of there.

In total, the 101 promise adds up to a rounded, complete view of you and your weight, looking at ways to eat, ways to cheat, ways to dress, what to ditch and why you should thank your stars that you live in an age of Solution Lingerie. The journey will be positive, enjoyable, progressive, arriving at a place where you are happier and stronger, freed from the shackles of thin and the torments of dieting.

In short, a 'diet' isn't just about what you (don't) eat; it's not vacuum-packed. It's about you, the whole you and how you feel about yourself. Start understanding this, and you're on the way to figuring it out. Ready?

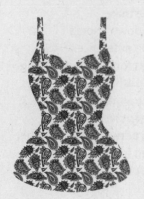 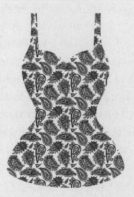 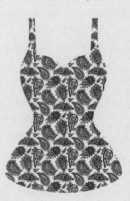

CHAPTER ONE
CHANGE YOUR MIND TO CHANGE YOUR SHAPE
Body Brilliance Starts in Your Head

First things first: do not stop eating! Isn't that a relief? But you *do* need to start loving – not that pretty cupcake, not those great ankle boots with the stack heel, not J Lo's new fringe, but YOURSELF. Your head needs to be in the right place from the outset. So get it out of the sand (or out of the fridge – or, come to that, out of that glossy magazine) and look in the mirror. This is where your journey begins; a little love and a lot of honesty will be your outriders on the road to glory. This chapter is about reassessing your relationship with the world. It's about seeing sense, gaining perspective and understanding what works for YOU. Not the girl in the lemon-yellow sweatpants. But you.

1 DON'T READ DIET BOOKS*

It is a dispiriting fact that the greatest preoccupation of our age is with weight and its loss. As the world grows ever richer and rounder, we seem to grow ever more fascinated by the heft or otherwise of our fellow men. Though, of course, we're far more interested in the women.

Think about how dieting and all its attendant nonsense have saturated our culture. How much time and effort it absorbs. We have trained ourselves to size people up in the blink of an eye. We're constantly aware of weight – its cruel lack or its licentious excess. We're hooked on A-list eating patterns, on quick-fix pills, on self-help miracle cures and the latest celebrity-endorsed regimes to issue from LA.

This, dear friends, is Diet Porn, a perverse phenomenon which undermines us all at a critical, visceral level. It gnaws away at our self-esteem, and sucks up vast tracts of time and energy which could be usefully expended elsewhere. While other eras basked in the Renaissance, the Golden Age, the Belle Epoque, we're lucky enough to have a TV schedule which boasts *Back Inside Britain's Fattest Man*. Look, I'm not expecting us to spend our evenings ruminating upon the complexities of our existence. But a little bit of thought beyond Gastric Bands of the Stars would make for a pleasant change.

Among the first requirements, the platform upon which you will stand if you are really going to tackle the bagginess that has crept into your life, is to Think Straight. You *have* to rid yourself of the dysfunction that marks our modern dance with diets. It's a ludicrous, exhausting gavotte and it has to stop. You have to be in the right frame of mind. You have to sidestep the weird extravagances, the wild promises, the wicked propaganda of an industry dedicated to keeping you in its grasp.

So stop staring at Jordan's butt and wondering how she does it. Start living. Stop measuring yourself against a warped societal norm. Start enjoying what you've got. Stop believing quick-fire fibs and what Susie Orbach calls 'the fictions that dominate our culture'. Start reading something edifying instead. Get your sustenance from poetry, from Plato, from dancing the tango in T-bar shoes, a red rose clenched between your teeth. Just don't get it from cake.

*This, I hasten to add, is not a diet book. It is a 'not-a-diet' book, designed to develop positive relationships – with your jeans, your butter dish, your waist, your world.

2 BELIEVE THAT YOU ARE BEAUTIFUL

You are already gorgeous. You just don't know it yet. To truly absorb this fundamental fact, you may well need to readjust your Fat Goggles and recognize that carrying a few extra pounds is not a cardinal sin, no matter what the more pernicious quarters of the media would have you believe. Dr Kerry Halliday, a psychologist specializing in body-shape issues, regularly encounters women who are a perfectly normal, decent size – 'and yet they've convinced themselves that a size 12 is fat! So many of the people I see are a healthy weight, but they have a fat head, full of fat thoughts. There's this constant dialogue of guilt. It's there when they go to sleep, it's there when they wake up, it's internal and introvert and isolating.'

Enough already! Embark on the new-you project from a position of STRENGTH. Loving yourself doesn't make you a narcissist, it makes you a realist, armed and ready to resist the onslaught of our bizarre, thin-obsessed culture.

You do, however, need to be realistic about your expectations. I've known for years that I'll never be a size 8, far less a size zero. I know that Kate Moss can do hot pants and I can't, that my thighs sometimes kiss in the middle like old friends, that a miniskirt makes me look like a maxi-pack . . . There's something very liberating about recognizing these small facts, about accepting them, and then – wahey – letting them go, like so many shiny helium balloons. You're suddenly free.

This doesn't mean letting *yourself* go, though. This project is not about giving in and giving up, installing yourself in the shadows and waiting for the seasons to change. No. This is a plan of action, a quest for change, a manifesto to celebrate all that is great about being a woman.

So accept yourself, right now. Don't live the dream, live the reality. You're not Katie Holmes. You have a soft tummy. You wish you looked better in a bikini. Watch those shiny balloons go, one by one. Pretty soon, you won't even know they were there. And remember all the while that the fat-cat dieting industry is founded upon the expectation of failure; you, my dear, should start with the bracing power of hope.

3 OPEN YOUR EYES AND RECOGNIZE YOUR WORTH

By and large – unless you have some karmic reason to believe otherwise – you only get one body. It may wax and wane, ebb and flow, but broadly speaking you're lumbered with these legs, that chest, those buttocks, this mortal coil. Rather than poke it in the eye with a fork, wouldn't it be better to love it? Just a bit? But how can you love someone you don't really know?

Before the off, you need to understand exactly what shape you're in. Unless you turn on the lights now, you'll never grasp the truth – so get a grip. Sneak a look. You won't bite. I'm not expecting you to conduct a microscopic investigation of every inch, but you do need to have a handle on how you really look, who you really are and whether those wide-legged palazzo pants are really such a good idea.

So stop ignoring your reflection – in shop windows, in the mirror, in those brutal changing rooms where you catch a rare glimpse of your unfamiliar buttocks . . . None of it is going anywhere unless you do. Look through holiday photos. Don't shy away from the truth – it's never as bad as you expect (though that bikini in Tenerife really was a shocker).

Once you have had a proper gawp – yes, naked, with the lights on – you can start to weigh up your options. I don't suggest you install vast mirrors on every available surface – you're not Peter Stringfellow – but do administer a good dose of exceptional honesty. If you're the kind of person who likes to keep scrapbooks and ticket stubs from amazing journeys, you might want to take 'before' photos so that you can marvel at the 'after' shots in a couple of months' time (best keep these to yourself).

Whatever you see, don't be mirror-miserable. If you face the music and feel fat, don't spiral off on a project of shame and finger-pointing. You're only on Point 3. We've barely begun! Instead of seeking out and dwelling on the downers, look for and big up your positive points, remembering all the while that you're never as fat as you feel. Your task – with the help of the next ninety-eight tips – is to stop feeling fat and start feeling fabulous. Understand now (and recall often as you read the next ten chapters) that a gentle softness, a Rubens roundness, is feminine and beautiful and *absolutely* fine. It is infinitely more appealing than a desperate yearning for a flat stomach and toothpick thighs. If in doubt, ask a man.

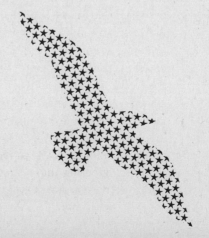

SHIFT YOUR SHAPE, NOT YOUR WEIGHT

It's worth noting early on that you – yes, *you* – don't really want to lose weight at all. What you want is to *change shape*. If you are round and bottom-heavy, you want to be leaner. If you are wide and wobbly, you want to be taut and toned. I know, I understand. Me too. The issue, then, isn't how much you weigh per se. It's not even your BMI rating. This score (mine happens to be 21.9) is necessarily abstract, a general theory that cannot hope to measure the particulars and peculiarities of the individual. It takes no account of body type, ethnicity or composition – and as such ought to be treated with informed caution. A perfectly fit, lean athlete can easily be classed as obese using this system. According to the BMI standard (your weight in kilograms divided by your height in metres squared) Brad Pitt is classed as technically 'overweight', while Arnold Schwarzenegger and George Clooney are both 'clinically obese'. Even Dame Kelly Holmes clocks in as a heavyweight.

If you're seriously overweight, or desperate to have a number stamped on your size, a BMI score may be of use to you – indeed there is no real alternative that does the job any better. But for a run-of-the-mill, slightly-on-the-chubby-side subject, knowing your BMI is about as much use as knowing how to do quadratic equations. And when did you last have to remember that the highest power of x is x^2?

Far better to feel the real. Use your eyes. Use your pants. Use your unforgiving and not-entirely-kind mirror. We all know, for instance, that muscle weighs more than fat. We all know that fat located in certain areas is more troublesome to the eye than in others. We all know that one woman's eleven-stone hell is another's eleven-stone paradise. Find your happy place.

4 STOP WORSHIPPING THIN AND LOVE THE SKIN YOU'RE IN

It is hardly a revelation to note that as a society we are obsessed to the point of distraction by thin – associating it, as a recent survey found, with 'success'. By the tender age of six, most girls are dissatisfied with their bodies and want to be thinner, according to research published in the *British Journal of Developmental Psychology*, with almost half believing they need to go on a diet to lose weight. 'Girls seemed particularly aware of teasing and likeability on the basis of weight and shape,' the report concludes. The psychologists' explanation of this body-bashing is that in these egalitarian times, given few remaining hierarchies based on religion, background, money or education, we tend to judge people in terms of their appearance. Image is currency. It's diverting to think that until the seventies, only overweight women dieted. Today, only overweight women don't.

Of course, this book is all about stopping that rot. While there's nothing sinister or odd about wanting to feel fit, be healthy and look great in a pair of shorts, there is danger in persuading yourself that all your troubles could be eliminated if only you slimmed down. Life – fat, thin or somewhere in between – will always pelt off on its own trajectory whether you are ten stone nine or eight stone nothing. Even at your gotta-be weight, you'll still have to deal with your husband/teenagers/ aggravating mother-in-law. There will still be bills and traffic jams and that annoying stain on the rug where you spilled red wine. You won't enter nirvana as your scales strike nine. So stop putting all your hopes and dreams into one skinny little packet. Recognize that being thin is not the same as having a good body. Know that thin can be thick (it won't make you bright; in fact, starving your body of essential nutrients is plain dumb). Once you've gained perspective, you'll probably lose weight. Life's weird like that.

USE YOUR BRAIN, NOT YOUR FORK

Kooky as it sounds, you can 're-programme' your brain to eat well. Along with physiological demands, hormone surges and social pressures, there is another influence at work on your appetite. Psychology.

The human mind is a lot like the human child. Tell it not to do something, deprive it of something (anything, really – *High School Musical* stickers, Spiderman lunch-boxes, chocolate-coated Brazil nuts), and it will want it *more than any other little thing on the face of the earth*. It will obsess. Ever tried to think 'I mustn't have that cake'? About as successful as 'I mustn't think of pink elephants,' right?

In a study by psychologists at the University of Hertfordshire, dieting was actually found to *increase* cravings for 'forbidden' foods such as chocolate. In their experiment, researchers showed eighty-five women a series of images of enticing chocolate cakes and oozy puddings drenched in fudge sauce – and found that subjects showed significantly more desire for these than when they were shown pictures of other covetable objects, such as perfume or Mercedes cars. So far, so what? Well, among *dieting* women (those who had dieted in the last year or who were on a diet at the time), the responses were even stronger. They experienced heightened cravings and feelings of guilt. 'Dieting appears to make a difference to how people perceive food, in this particular instance, chocolate,' the study concluded. 'Instead of helping people to eat more healthily and to cut down on products which are bad for their health, the negative effect induced by dieting appears to have the opposite effect in that it can increase the desire for the actual foods they are trying to avoid . . . If we constantly deprive the brain of the food we most desire we crave it even more.'

Clearly, you need to nip that right in the bud – first by allowing yourself just a little of what you fancy, and then by moderating your behaviour around foods that will make you fat. As it turns out, 'think thin' is not such an empty phrase. According to another recent report, it *is* possible to think yourself thinner. The study involved forty-seven women who were each asked to spend half an hour thinking after having consumed a large lunch (something I've always found delightfully easy to do, though falling asleep is a constant threat). Researchers found that encouraging the subjects to remember the details of their last meal made them a third less likely to eat snacks. Suzanne Higgs, who led the research, submits that this could point to a stronger connection between memory and body weight than previously thought. 'How well people can remember could be a factor in explaining why some eat more than others,' she told the *Daily Telegraph*. 'There are certain things that we do now which are rather distracting and could stop people recalling quite as well what they have eaten.'

So pay attention. Watch what you eat, in a non-invasive, laid-back sort of way – like a chilled parent keeping an unseen eye on their kid in a paddling pool. Some people uncover the truth by keeping a food diary, believing that detailing their intake limits it and helps avoid 'unconscious eating'. Try it. It doesn't work for me. I did once write a food log covering the period between breakfast and lunch – and found the experience so tedious that I turned to shortbread for solace and to add texture to my day. But it may work for you. The idea, really, is to be conscious of what you eat and know where your foibles lie, waiting to trip you up at the first tummy rumble.

Even if you don't buy the psychobabble, you can at least recognize that your ego, super-ego and id need to be pulling in the same direction, towards a healthy, balanced, confident new you. You'll do way better if you stop punishing yourself about your body and the space it occupies. Punishment will only lead to rebellion and a recidivist streak, hurling you senseless back towards the open fridge. Be kind. Think good thoughts (but don't add fudge sauce).

FAT DAYS MAKE YOU HUMAN,
NOT HUMONGOUS

You know how it feels. You wake up all wrong. Your face stares bleakly out from the mirror, demanding to know why you even bothered emerging from the sack. Your wardrobe is a freakish obstacle course, a land of booby traps and trip-wires, filled with oddly shaped jackets and cheek-sapping colours. That dress you looked a-*mazing* in last Friday? Nightmare. The sexy, sultry siren shoes? Slutty. The red V-neck sweater, the one that made you feel like Gina Lollobrigida? More like what-a-load-of-crapida.

There are days when the very same clothes on the very same body can feel inordinately different – and it all depends on something as insubstantial and subjective as your mood. We all have days like these. No one is immune to bad-hair days, bad-skin days, big-bum days, days that are full of ladders and scuffs, broken nails and dashed dreams. They arise because we're human.

More to the point, they arise because we're women.

They're the brute consequence of hormones, emotions, perception, a chance comment, an off look. These unfathomables can't be put in a Petri dish and prodded with a pipette. They can't be marshalled into a thesis to be delivered at a symposium. But they can have a potent effect on your day and how you feel about it. Accept them. Don't fight them. Today will become tomorrow, and that dress that makes you look like a pumpkin may have turned you into a princess by then, just because you've *changed your mind*. Even Hamlet knew that 'there is nothing either good or bad, but thinking makes it so'. Don't read too much into it. Read Shakespeare instead.

6 LAUGH IN THE FACE OF CELEBRITY MAGAZINES

Open any weekly magazine and you'll come across the usual parade of whip-thin women, their brows set in grim determination to avoid lunch. Over the past decade, many of our contemporary heroines seem to have reduced like stock on a stove until there's nothing left of them. Nothing but skin and bones. It is this look, this *lack*, that has become an aspiration and inspiration for a whole generation of girls.

We've always admired icons, of course. Jennifer Aniston herself remembers idolizing actresses as a child. 'Their hair, their clothes, their make-up were perfect,' she says. 'Looking back, I realize it wasn't a good thing. I was wanting to become this unattainable person.' The consequence, she later confessed, was an eating disorder that wrecked her health. 'I started taking vitamins and exercising and went too far. You get into that Zone Diet thing and you kind of get addicted to that.' Similarly, Sarah Michelle Gellar has let slip that being a celebrity means inhabiting another space, another dimension – and that for a civilian to join in the charade is a hopeless enterprise. 'Look,' she says, 'it's crazy for people to try to be as thin as we are. We have personal trainers and personal chefs. It's our job to look this way.'

Clearly, there's no point even attempting to keep up with the weightless A-list – though many mere mortals, seeing the absence of proper female flesh up there on the pedestal of fame, will try. I've known this truth for years, of course – ever since, well over a decade ago, I stumbled upon the art director of *Vogue* magazine using a scalpel to carve a few centimetres off Claudia Schiffer's ankles. It was, I hasten to add, a transparency he was working on, not Schiffer herself, which would have made an awful mess of the parquet floor. But even so, I have always been pretty miffed that even Claudia – an original supermodel and all-round babe – wasn't deemed quite good enough for public consumption in her natural state.

In real life, of course, celebrities have to work their butts off (literally) to look even halfway gorgeous. If they ever stopped making an almighty effort, everything would collapse, like a lolly left out in the sun. I promise you. With all the preening, pummelling and priming that goes on, it's little wonder that most of them don't speak a second language, make their own marmalade or play the piccolo. They simply don't have the time.

They do, however, have the time to follow zany diets based on spirulina, bee pollen and obscure Amazonian berries unavailable on the open market. It's all cayenne-pepper cordials and Myoplex Protein Shakes out there in the Hollywood Hills. Fridges are locked at night and the key sent home with the housekeeper. Trainers are on the doorstep at dawn, armed with grape-seed extract and the latest in high-tensile exercise apparatus.

'Clearly, there's no point even attempting to keep up with the weightless A-list – though many mere mortals will try.'

Sure, the bodies these women end up with are, very often, stupendous. But at what cost? Not long ago, an engaging picture turned up showing the chance meeting of Cameron Diaz and Victoria Beckham at the MTV Music Awards. Both had poured their syrup-coloured selves into tiny little tubes which were, briefly, doing duty as dresses. At one end of the dress, the women were all naked neck and shoulder blade, taut face and bronzed skin, their breasts buns of steel. At the other end of operations, both wore silver winkle-pickers, which looked like the kind of implements Gordon Ramsay uses to kill crabs. This, it struck me, is the modern uniform for celebrity dress-up. Perfect skin, muscular boobs, long limbs, wicked heels. And a body primed like an F1 piston, in such a streamlined state that its maintenance would clearly be a full-time, staff-required, no-let-up job.

Such extreme maintenance has lately become the stock lifestyle in Hollywood and beyond, leaving folk like us languishing in the slow lane. Bombarded daily by images of physical perfection, we've come to view these bionic women as normal. And so, while our glossy magazines are populated almost entirely by sparrow-models and syrup-skinned celebrities, the back pages are dedicated to fat-busting fad diets, liposuction ads and essays on why five-bite meals will turn you into a Glamazon in a lunch hour (as long as you don't actually have any lunch).

In the process, many of us have lost all perspective, developing unnatural ideas about what women are supposed to look like. Think of our screen stars, our popstars, any model on any catwalk anywhere in the world – I've got handbags which weigh more than they do. I could fold someone like Lindsay Lohan up and stash her in my pocket. In this Looking Glass world, a ninety-pounder is a heavyweight. True perspective can be gained when you consider that the pin-up of the 1890s was Lillian Russell, all *two hundred pounds of her*. We don't even have to mention Jayne Mansfield, Rita Hayworth, Jane Russell, Sophia Loren, Raquel Welch – none of whom would get the job today – to know that something's up.

To maintain this abnormal body shape, our icons – those brave enough to step up to the plate and admit it – are permanently hungry. Elizabeth Hurley has admitted as much. Marcia Cross, who plays Bree Van De Kamp in *Desperate Housewives*, recently confessed that staying thin was 'a living hell', and that she felt she had been banned from eating since joining the show. Actresses, models, singers, presenters – all are subject to the dictatorship of thin enforced by the minders, agents and producers who know very well what sells. It happened to All Saints, to Girls Aloud, to Myleene Klass. I know from my experience in the fashion industry that it happens to hopeful young girls from the moment that first Polaroid is taken in the reception of the modelling agency. Christina Ricci recalls the favoured put-down for wannabe actresses in Hollywood: 'They say "She looks too healthy", which means "She needs to lose weight".'

It's a strong current, this grim undertow of the image game, and it's almost impossible to resist. Some try. When British model of the moment Daisy Lowe arrived in New York for her first season of shows, she was called 'a little hefty'. Her response? 'I am who I am. My old agents in New York suggested I lose weight. So I moved agents. I'm extremely proud of the fact that I am two sizes bigger than most models. Being a stick is so unsexy.'

Too right, and it's something that magazine editors are slowly, gingerly, coming to realize. Says Sophia Neophitou-Apostolou, editor of *10* magazine: 'The designers I work with now are demanding a more womanly girl and art directors are complaining that, these days, they're adding curves rather than shaving them off.' Those art directors do, however, want those curves in the regulation sex-pot places, as Elizabeth Hurley recently discovered when her breasts were electronically enlarged for the cover of *Cosmopolitan* magazine. 'On my last *Cosmo* cover,' she told *Details*, 'they added about five inches to my breasts. It's very funny. I have, like, massive knockers. Huge. Absolutely massive.'

Right. So let's just admit that it's a weird, air-brushed world in the inner sanctum of fame. You, however, are not an inflatable doll, to be pumped up and down at will. Your challenge is to ignore these extremes and reacquaint yourself with the bell-curve of normal womanly weight. Real women are soft in places, good to cuddle. If the celebrity template starts to look reasonable to your eye, then stop staring. Shut the magazine. Go for a jog instead.

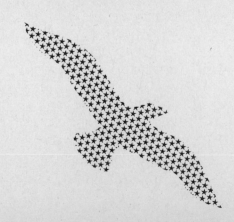

THE SIGH OF SIZE:
HOW WE LOST OUR WAY

Twenty-five years ago, the average model weighed 8 per cent less than the average woman (yes, Twiggy was abnormally petite in her day). Today's model weighs 23 per cent less than the average.

As long ago as 2000, the BMA, in its report *Eating Disorders, Body Image and the Media*, noted that the extreme thinness of celebrities was 'both unachievable and biologically inappropriate', observing that the gap between the media ideal and reality appeared to be making eating disorders worse. 'At present, certain sections of the media provide images of extremely thin or underweight women in contexts which suggest that these weights are healthy or desirable,' it stated, recommending that normal women in the upper reaches of a healthy weight should be 'more in evidence on television as role models for young women'. Television producers and those in advertising should review their employment of very thin women, and the Independent Television Commission should review its advertising policy, the report recommended. Almost a decade on, the opposite has happened.

Every now and again, one of their own takes up arms. Emma Thompson, for example, is known to be on a crusade against the idiocy of thin that plagues her profession – and has intervened when Kate Winslet (on the set of *Sense and Sensibility*) and Haley Atwell (on *Brideshead Revisited*) were encouraged by producers to shrink a couple of sizes. But generally speaking, it's a way of life in which many are either trapped or complicit.

It is perhaps worth regaining a little perspective about what constitutes beauty. Back in 1913, *Webster's Dictionary* defined the word thus: 'properties pleasing the eye, the ear, the intellect, the aesthetic faculty or the moral sense'. Hmm. I'm not sure that a double-zero perma-hungry woman with a lock on her fridge door fits any of those criteria. Are you?

FIND YOUR STRENGTH AND PLAY TO IT

While our forebears occupied themselves with the knotty issues of universal suffrage and how to feed a family of seven on a single turnip, we lucky, lazy twenty-first-century women spend a very great deal of time pondering our own navels. A recent survey in *Grazia* magazine uncovered quite how spectacularly our bodies dominate our lives. Seven out of ten of us apparently think life would improve greatly if we had a 'good' body (ach, world peace is so passé); half of us think that our body shape and size spoils our sex life (although most men would probably beg to differ; as Phil Hilton, ex-editor of lads' mag *Nuts*, once admitted on the subject of perfect boobs: 'Men think all breasts are good and are delighted to have access to any at all. The idea that they are connoisseurs is inaccurate').

Yet most women – and it matters little how educated, successful or, indeed, beautiful we are – despair about arms which wobble, chins which double and thighs which meet in the middle. Rather than find our strengths, we are continually on the lookout for weakness – the sweat-stain on the shirt, the spinach in the teeth, the cellulite clambering out of the cab.

Leeds Medical School psychologist Dr Andrew Hill believes that disliking particular body parts in this piecemeal, picky way is a modern phenomenon. 'Now we have the technology to change specific areas of the body,' he says. 'We can be more hypercritical simply because we can fix the problem. It's all part of the new culture of self-improvement which wasn't around thirty years ago.'

And so we chip away, undermining our own confidence, sinking our own ship. The point is that we *all* have our unbecoming bits, the stuff we'd prefer to keep under wraps. Madonna, for instance, despises her chubby 'Italian' thighs, inherited from her mother; Erin O'Connor has a complex about her 'Celtic knees'; Nadine Coyle of Girls Aloud can't stomach her legs ('I look at them sometimes and want to throw up,' she says); George Michael's face is always pictured half in shadow because he doesn't like the other half.

Lily Allen, for one, is learning to deal. She worked out long ago how to capitalize on her assets, generally wearing prom dresses to hide what she considers to be her substantial caboose: 'My favourite feature is my waist,' she says. 'It's always been tiny. My thighs aren't tiny and that's why I started wearing dresses. I was conscious of my big bum and thighs, and I discovered dresses hid them.'

'Madonna, despises her chubby "Italian" thighs, inherited from her mother; Erin O'Connor has a complex about her "Celtic knees"; Nadine Coyle of Girls Aloud can't stomach her legs.'

It is Kelly Osbourne, though, who has mastered the art of strength-playing. 'I would never want to be perfect,' she smiles (and, yes, you *know* she's smiling). 'I like the fact that I have round bits and will probably always be a bit fat. I don't want to be perfect, I want to be an individual ... Recently, for the first time in my life I actually put on a dress and thought, "You look beautiful." It was a Belville Sassoon dress that I wore to an awards ceremony and I spent a good twenty minutes looking at myself in the mirror thinking, "I never, ever thought you would look like this."'

Don't you just love that? Don't you want to give her a hug? Buy her a hot chocolate (skinny, no cream)? Now then. On a personal note, seeing as we're all sharing, I'd like to introduce my not-quite-but-almost-perfect ankles. I got them genetically, along with a good ear, a decent singing voice and a nose that gives generous shade on a hot day. So I wear fancy shoes, cropped trousers, lots of dresses, giving these ankles a lead role in my life, in the knowledge that while they're dancing centre stage, my less excellent regions can fade unheeded into the background. My middle, for instance.

I am one of those women with a soft centre. My stomach is squashy and yielding, like a warm bun, though resolutely stubborn in its refusal to budge despite the occasional desperate burst of sit-ups, curls and the odd stern talking-to. It is my *bête noire* and bugbear, this belly of mine. It makes me feel as if I'm carrying someone else's shopping (Look! No hands!). But have I mentioned my fabulous ankles . . .?

See? Take a tip. You may loathe your shoulders, knees or toes (though I'll put good money on it being belly, boobs or bottom). But before you start prodding yourself with the vicious little stick of self-hatred, find the bit you love the most. Not the least. The *most*. If it's calves, show them. If it's cleavage, take the plunge. Don't point out your thunderous thighs and donate ammunition to your adversaries; big up your pretty wrists, those full lips, that smile. Believe in your beauty, don't fixate on your foibles. If you can make the best of your bummers with the judicious use of candlelight and prom dresses, then so much the better.

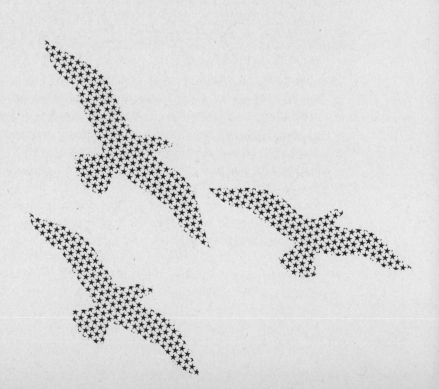

IT'S YOUR BODY, BUDDY ...
HOW TO NEUTRALIZE THE NEGATIVES

* **Heavy in the hips?** Well, so was Sophia Loren in her heyday. The trick here is to go for the cling, making a fuss of your bust and whittling away at the waist, just like Lily Allen does, for that classic hourglass appeal.

* **Blocky in the shoulder?** Try a wrap, a plunge neck, a killer cleavage. It's how Jessica Alba and Helen Mirren get by, poor dears.

* **Short in the leg?** A boot-cut with a kick in the hem, a skirt which stops dead at the knee, a neat short-line jacket to lengthen a leg ... all will help to stretch your proportions and add an illusory lift. It goes without saying that heels are your loyal ally. Kylie in flats? I don't think so.

* **Piggy in the middle?** *Me too!* You don't need a tummy tuck, you need a tummy tamer, one of the many practical ways to scoot diplomatically over the issue. So, drop your waistband or raise it to the empire line; choose tops with a forgiving swing in the hem, or firm tailoring to keep you safely tucked in.

* **Broad in the beam?** Doesn't keep Beyoncé and J Lo off the map. Go an inch or two wider at the shoulder and the hem to make your waist work harder.

We'll expand on these issues – and dozens more – in Chapters Five and Seven, where you'll discover exactly how to dress to play up your personal positives. Before we do the detail, though, you need to grasp a basic ...

8 DISCOVER YOUR OWN STYLE

What you wear is of absolute import and impact, your passport
to a whole world of thin. For every questionable bubble skirt,
for every dodgy poncho in the 'must-have colour of the season',
there's a piece of clothing that will make your body sing, simply
because it nails your own unique presence, your sense of self. This,
incidentally, may have very little to do with the trends of the day.
Discovering clothes which work *with* you rather than fight against
you is the fundamental principle of great style, and the linchpin
of weight-loss dressing.

It's not just what you wear, but how you wear it that matters.
It's in the tilt of a hat, the nonchalant throw of a scarf, the purpose
in a stride; it's about risking a clash (it never did Yves Saint Laurent
any harm), or perfecting a classic (a tux for evening? Go for it.
A cashmere crew? There are very good reasons why these superior
staples have been loved for so long). Everything you climb into
gives out subtle signals, coded impressions that can captivate or
caress a room. Or turn it off like a switch. Your mission is to convey
a message of confidence. Ease. By the time you reach Point 101,
I can guarantee that you'll have this self-possession, this poise,
stashed in your pocket like a lucky charm.

For the moment, you need to know that, like much in modern
life, it's all in the sell. Walk into that room like you own it, or at
the very least like it owes you. Behavioural psychologist Sue Firth
agrees that style is the consequence of confidence – available to
anyone of any age and any shape willing to make the effort. 'It is
about time-taking,' she says, 'about attention to detail. The whole
impression sends out a message of charisma, and that is what
we are drawn to. Projecting style is a function of confidence,
self-esteem and self-respect.'

Rather than trying to find the silhouette of the season, try
to find your *style*. Be true to you. As Quentin Crisp had it: 'Fashion
is what you adopt when you don't know who you are.' So, if that
competitively on-trend sweater is making your chest look like a
sack of ferrets, ditch it. If the catwalk calls for white trousers and

your tush calls for mercy, give it a break. If you always get compliments in that subtle grey trouser suit, the one you've had for years, the one which adores you, regardless, like a faithful hound? Wear it, whatever the catwalk has to say on the matter. Don't be in thrall to fashion – instead, hum gently to yourself that just because it's in, it won't make you thin. As Ingrid Bergman wisely said, 'Be yourself. The world worships an original.' One of the best ways to do this is to . . .

9 DEVELOP YOUR TRADEMARK LOOK

A few months back, over coffee, my great friend Carla went through something of an existential *crise*, right here in my kitchen. 'Who am I? Who AM I?' she wailed, head in hands and one strand of hair (I couldn't help but notice) dangling perilously close to the cold coffee at her elbow.

'Ah, Carla,' I said in my least patronizing tone, 'as you get a tiny bit older, you can no longer fanny about with toy-town trends, changing your haircut every third minute and expecting your body to settle into dungarees or plus-fours just because Marc Jacobs tells you to. No. What you need, as you age, is a Thing.'

'A Thing?'

The congress of cold coffee and hair was now complete, and Carla was dabbing at the result with a Handy Andy.

'Yep. A Thing. Like Grace Coddington has all that fabulous red hair. And Issy Blow wore hats shaped like *Apollo 13* or deep-sea crustacea. Victoria Beckham does all those wicked dresses which fit tighter than skin, and Anna Wintour has her blow-dry, and . . . You need to find yourself to project yourself.'

I was quite chuffed with this little epigram, but Carla seemed unimpressed. She sniffed loudly into the caffeinated tissue.

'But what's *my* Thing?'

'Go monochrome,' I suggested brightly.

This is always my best advice to the lost sheep on the fashion farm. It's a tip I picked up years ago, when working alongside a particular fashion editor. Like all top-of-the-range stylists, this woman had access to almost anything her heart could desire. Trunks of Dior, towers of Versace, truck-loads of Armani. Rhinestones, cashmere, wild silks from Samarkand, snakeskin handbags, Gucci shoes, Pucci pants. And what did she choose?

Black trousers, white shirt. Every day. Religiously. She had obviously taken a vow, quite early on in her career, to 'throw a look' – a look, it has to be said, which owed more than a nod to the Einstein school of dressing (he kept seven identical suits in the closet and wore them in strict rotation, thus allowing his brain to settle on more taxing topics than whether blue and green should ever be seen).

This particular editor worked at the magazine every day in black pumps, exquisitely cut coal-black trousers and the kind of shirt which would glow in the dark, so clean and pin-fresh was its whiteness. She always looked immaculate (I suspect she changed into an identical outfit after lunch, or whenever someone sneezed near her, or opened a purse). There was none of that dizzy wheeling about in search of the next big trend; she did that for a living, so her own wardrobe simply maintained a calm decorum. It helped that she was gamine and adorable to look at, but her approach would pretty much suit anyone of a certain age who knows that her dolly days are over.

Finding your Thing bestows upon you a sense of arrival, a feeling of strength and self-awareness. It feels like coming home. After much deliberation, Carla and I divined her Thing. Turns out she's a jingly jewellery sort of girl. She's going to wear charming bracelets which chime and chink as she walks, set against a blank canvas of jeans, white T-shirts and well-cut, expensive trouser suits. Genius, I think you'll agree.

No need to go mad, you see. Your signature could be something simple and chic (diamond studs, a slash of red lipstick) or something quirky and cool (trainers with your prom dress, a beehive with your ballet shoes, a bit of gilt and a lot of kohl). Personally, until I hit thirty-eight I was all tawny hair and push-up bra. More lately, it's French navy, a becoming shade of teal and an aquamarine ring that could double as an offensive weapon. For you, it may be the trench, or the tailoring of Savile Row. It may be corsage and corsetry, or a crisp fitted shirt and bangles to the elbow. Whatever it is, find it. Wear it. Often. Not always. But often. Be remembered – the woman in white, the lady in red, the one most likely to succeed. Think of Diana Vreeland's rings, Katharine Hepburn's trousers, Coco Chanel's bouclé jackets, camellias and pearls. If in doubt, find your icon – Monroe, Stefani, Jolie, Winfrey – and copy her. Style-jacking your heroine is no sin. It's the very axis of intelligent dressing. If Karl Lagerfeld can do it, then you can too.

Don't, however, set your signature in aspic and wait for death. Let it evolve, sticking to the general trajectory, but taking in the view along the way. Developing a Look, you'll soon find, is like developing armour; whatever the slings and arrows chucked at you, you're safe.

WHO TO HIJACK:
TOP CELEBRITY STYLE STAPLES

A trademark fashion staple is a little like having a PA you can trust, or your own eyebrowist who understands the ins and outs of your face. They can draw attention to your fabulous bits, or run interference for your dodgy bits. Think for a moment about the inhabitants of the world's 'best-dressed' lists and you'll soon see that a signature is very often the element that marks them out from the gormless masses. The trick is to find – or steal – a style and stick to it, a bit like:

✳ **Elizabeth Hurley's white jeans**. She's worn them through thin and thin – even when they were about as fashionable as a jab in the eye with a kipper tie. 'I probably own thirty pairs,' Hurley admits. 'I love it and I know it works.' Elizabeth is, of course, glossy and groomed enough to make white jeans look St Tropez chic rather than shopping-mall slappy. But why does she wear them all the time? Because they have a strong style message: 'I'm thin!' they cry, 'And rich! I dry clean!' White jeans may not be quite your cup of tea – so experiment until you discover exactly what is: Grey needlecords? Black velvet skinnies? Drill-cotton Capris? Take your pick, but make it *your own*. Stamp your style.

⭐ **Anna Wintour's classic bob and Chanel sunglasses**. If you are the most observed fashion plate on the planet – and, as editor of *Vogue*, how could you not be? – you need to tread confidently on the tightrope of style. Ms Wintour does so with consummate ease, chiefly by relying on a signature triumvirate of big, bad shades, dead-straight bob and hot-from-the-atelier haute couture. Like I said. Armour. I'm guessing your wardrobe is a little light on £28,000 couture frocks from Chanel – but a sleek haircut and a signature accessory? You can afford those.

⭐ **J Lo's hipster flares**. Lopez, as we all know, has a glorious Latina butt, and hipster flares are a way of putting it up there in lights. We've all been fascinated with that rump for years; it's J Lo's USP. The trademark trousers maximize attention on those buttocks, and – thanks to the additional material dancing about at ground level – have a pneumatic appeal, exaggerating curves and generally looking *grrrr*eat (it works for flamenco dancers, too).

⭐ **Kate Moss's Very Important Pieces**. Consider what makes Kate's wardrobe tick: the Ossie Clark coats, the vintage rock 'n' roll jackets once worn by Keith Moon and bought at auction, the thirties nightgowns, the statement jewellery that talks a helluva lot more than she does. For all her style dipping, Kate is remarkably constant. She relies on quality not quantity, buying originals not knock-offs, authentic, timeless pieces not poppy trends. She invariably attends business meetings in a Chanel power suit, 'like Jackie O,' she says, 'but with a T-shirt, a power watch from Rolex and my Vivienne Westwood Sex shoes'. Her favourite shop is S. J. Phillips, a jeweller on New Bond Street, which she visits every birthday; over the years, it has become a cornerstone of her Look. The point here is that she doesn't patrol the fashion landscape hoovering up the latest bits of fluff to tumble off a catwalk. She knows her brand and sticks with it, occasionally flirting with a fringe or a new YSL handbag to keep us on our toes.

✳ **Elle Macpherson's blazer**. An anachronism, perhaps, but being tall, Elle has the ideal figure for the coolly classic blazer (let's face it, she has the ideal figure for a Sainsbury's carrier bag). A blazer is, though, a forgiving staple for *any* shape – a snappy, practical wardrobe workhorse that can look particularly hot if it's worn a shade too small (shove up the sleeves for extra sass appeal). If you're looking to copy Elle, steer clear of brass buttons and fire up your sober jacket with attitude; whatever mood you go for, avoid smart – you don't want to look like James Hewitt. But you do want to look a bit ACDC performing 'Highway to Hell' in front of a stadium audience.

✳ **Audrey Hepburn's Capri pants**. Cropped trousers – to the shin or the knee – are a good way to point up delicate ankles and show off a pair of coquettish pumps. They're cute, too. Ever since Capris first took off in the fifties, thanks to Audrey in *Sabrina* and *Funny Face*, the cropped trouser has suggested a carefree, run-along-the-beach sort of fashion freedom. If they could talk, they'd giggle and then smoke a cigarette (but not inhale).

Once you start to crack the code, you'll notice that most celebrities, past and present, have a Thing. Dita Von Teese? Red lips, corset. Jemima Khan? Floaty layers, wide hair. Bianca Jagger? Black suit, white shirt. Amanda Harlech? Vintage Chanel, vintage Dior. Judi Dench? Layers of linen. Jayne Mansfield? Turbo sweater. Annie Leibovitz? The woman in black. Daphne Guinness? Wicked tailoring and a flurry of feathers. You can spot her at fifty paces, which just about sums up my point.

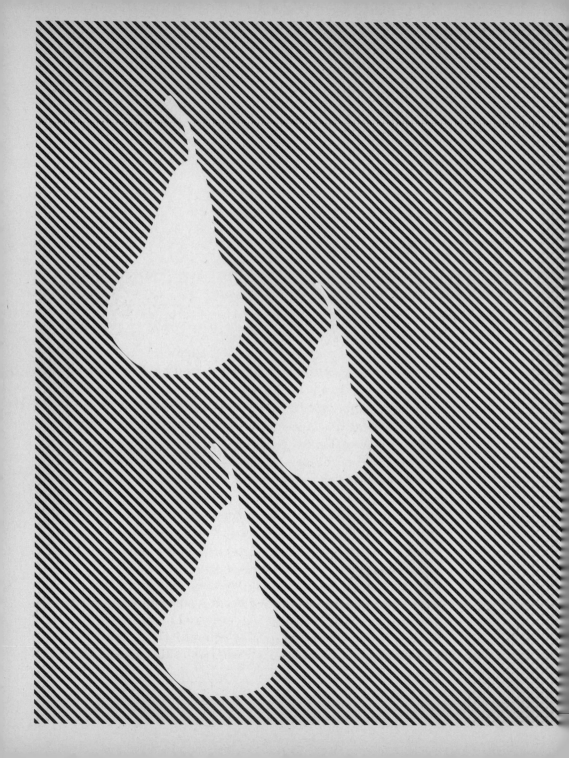

CHAPTER TWO
THE NO-DIET DOZEN
The Twelve-Step Programme to Fix Your Fattening Habits

You've read all the books, you've torn bits out of magazines and tried to subsist on a handful of raisins and a couple of mangetouts. Well, so have I. Having digested many a diet book on your behalf, I have identified the useful bits and put the rest out to compost. These, then, are your golden rules, the Twelve Steps that will whisk you from the dumpy ground floor to the soaring penthouse in the time it takes you to read this chapter. With the following pointers, you'll have the basics for a new and healthy relationship with your fridge; by Point 21, you'll be well on your way to body-love. As Voltaire put it, 'Nothing would be more tiresome than eating and drinking if God had not made them a pleasure as well as a necessity.' So prepare to eat *more*, not less (I told you this was a no-diet book). Here's how to uphold the pleasure principle without busting a gut.

10 EAT A DECENT BREAKFAST

Skipping meals is never clever. Think about it for a minute and you may be able to convince yourself that dropping breakfast will have you dropping a dress size. Tee hee, you'll think, no Weetabix this morning! That's saved me 250 calories and it's only three hours till lunch!

But think about it for *five* minutes and you'll soon realize that the opposite is true. The first thing you need to observe and understand is that you are an animal. Sorry, but you are. Deal with it. You have ancestors, sweetie. You, like me, started out in the primordial soup, and we're still carrying all the evolutionary baggage which got us out of there and into this incredible world of eyelash curlers and iPhones. This means that our bodies still respond to our environment in an age-old way and no amount of wheedling or needling will change the way they do business. As countless studies have shown, skipping a meal – or going on any variety of deprivation diet – merely evokes a primal 'fear of hunger' response, which will scupper any attempt you may make to lose weight. The brute biology of it all has been rehearsed in full elsewhere, but, in case you've been living under a tablecloth for years, I will give you a bullet-point meander through the basics:

✳ **In times of food deprivation** (for example, during the first desperate days of Atkins), the body's ancient hard-wiring kicks in.

✳ **Your body** – which really does have a mind of its own – decides it is being starved. Hmm, it thinks. No food. Where the devil will the next meal come from?

✳ **Hormones muster**. Worry not, they sing, we'll help you store some calories. We'll simply overrule the usual satiety signals, we'll sharpen up those hunger pangs. Trust us, we'll get you through this!

✳ **Anticipating further hardship and vicissitude**, your body goes into squirrel mode, storing more food as fat, and breaking down less of it as energy. It clings on for all it's worth and, hungry as

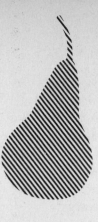

you may be, you'll *never* get to zip up that pencil skirt. This, let's face it, is not part of your game plan at all.

Unpredictable, unfulfilling or omitted meals make you *hang on to fat stores* in anticipation of the next period of food scarcity (whether it arrives or not). Thus, most of the guff you find in diet regimes will, by the laws of your very own body, backfire.

Further food for thought comes from a Nottingham University study which found that keeping meal patterns constant also has definite metabolic advantages – associated with a greater 'thermic' effect of food (the energy cost of its digestion and absorption), a lower energy intake and lower 'bad' cholesterol. For sustained weight loss, then, you need regular, reliable meals, best consumed in the following order:

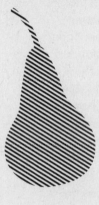

✳ **A good breakfast**. Breakfast kick-starts your metabolism, which has become sluggish and reluctant overnight, so it really ought to be the most important meal of the day, not just something you stuff in your face halfway between the shower and the station. In a five-year study of almost seven thousand men and women, researchers at Addenbrooke's Hospital in Cambridge found that those who ate the biggest breakfasts put on the least weight over a set period, despite consuming more food overall each day than those who ate sparingly in the mornings.

Cameron Diaz has taken this advice to heart and eats her dinner (garlicky lemon chicken with broccolini, since you ask) at breakfast time. Odd fish. But she says it keeps her going all day: 'I started doing it when I'd go surfing because I could go out for four hours and not get hungry.' Angelina Jolie did something similar to regain her killer shape after having twins. Her 'upside-down eating' involved a vast morning meal (a full English, apparently), with calorie consumption petering out over the course of the day, ending with a scant cup of homemade vegetable soup for supper.

You, however, might prefer to go to work on Madonna's much more prosaic secret diet food: a humble bowl of porridge. This dynamite dish guarantees to keep you feeling fuller longer, particularly after exercise or before taking on the Duke of

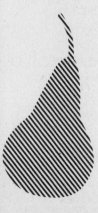

Cumberland at the Battle of Culloden. Slow-burning, space-filling oats are formidable little power flakes, the food of Zeus (they may even slow the ageing process, which is frankly too good a possibility to ignore).

While I'm all for porridge, it would help if you don't add demerara sugar, golden syrup, strawberry jam or any combination of the three. Train yourself to like it plain. Jumbo oats make it more interesting; skimmed milk will, of course, slim it right down. Even better, make your porridge with water, in fine Scottish tradition. If you really want to get into the thick of it, you could always entertain the Highland customs of the porridge pot (some say it should only ever be stirred in a clockwise direction, using the right hand, so as not to stir up the devil; others contend that porridge should be spoken of as 'they'. They, by the way, should be eaten standing up. With a bone spoon).

If porridge doesn't do it for you, go for a decent slow-release, low-sugar muesli. If you have both time and inclination, make your own, with oatflakes, chopped nuts, an assortment of interesting seeds and the zing of grated apple. If not, you can have it custom-mixed in Austria to your exact spec – adding Tibetan goji berries or taking out all the sultanas; find out more at mymuesli.com.

The idea of all this is to eat enough to preclude the need for a second breakfast at elevenish. You are not Winnie the Pooh. So, before you finish your porridge and start loading the dishwasher, one more tip: add protein. A recent study at Purdue University in Indiana found that eating a breakfast of eggs or bacon (or both) for breakfast elicited a greater sense of sustained fullness throughout the day, compared to eating protein for lunch or dinner. It's all in the timing. So add a slice of lean ham, a poached egg, a sliver of smoked salmon, green eggs and ham, a skewer of garlicky chicken – you decide – and it will set you right up for the day. Or at least until . . .

✳ **A protein-rich lunch**. By rights, this should be your main meal of the day – so don't waste the glory by settling for a second-rate sandwich and a slab of rocky road. Go to town. Make a meal of it. Linger. I like the Ayurvedic principle that we are designed to eat a larger meal in the middle of the day because our 'digestive fire' is strongest between ten a.m. and two p.m., allowing our system to operate at peak efficiency. You may think this is codswallop. Fine, but do try to eat lunch at *lunch* time, won't you? Leave it any later and studies show you are more likely to consume a greater number of calories. Do, however, bear in mind that glucose levels plummet in that post-lunch dip, so you might want to have a few nuts about your person for that mid-afternoon slip slot (I recommend almonds, as we'll see in Chapter Four).

✳ **A carb curfew after five p.m**. With the greatest respect to dear departed Dr Atkins, there *is* a time and a place for carbohydrates. Just not too many, the right, complex kinds, and not at supper. Why? Well . . . Some dieticians say that the body will burn fat only after it has first depleted its store of carbohydrates, so why make night carbs an obstacle? Others submit that our metabolism is on go-slow at night and will tend to store night carbs as body fat. Some women report less bloating when they reduce their night carbs. Whatever, whatever. The science isn't really sussed on this one quite yet. All you really need to know is that if you cut back on carbs in the evening, you are likely to diminish your overall daily calorie intake without it being too much of a sacrifice. If, by contrast, you down a twelve-inch pizza late at night, and then sleep on it? *Arrivederci* slim.

✳ **A smallish supper**. The idea here, really, is to go easy in the evening; as the irritating old saying goes, 'Breakfast for a king, lunch for a prince, dinner for a pauper.' The problem is that our culture, with its speedy days and lazier nights, its autopilot evening eating and its socially prescribed multi-course suppers, tends to 'backload' calories at the end of the day. If dining out, we'll bravely embark on an epic journey from appetizer to coffee, taking in whatever sorbets, savouries, side dishes and specials come our way, as if doing it for a bet. At home, we associate evenings with wallowing in food and drink, and if we weren't consuming, wouldn't we get a trifle . . . you know . . . *bored*?

'Evenings are the time when most people munch on high-fat foods, such as cakes and biscuits, because they are bored or tired,' says Louise Sutton, a senior lecturer in health and exercise science at Leeds Metropolitan University. OK. So, a carb curfew will put paid to that (eat a little more protein instead in the evening; it will help you stay fuller longer). And if you're plagued by the soul-rotting ennui of an evening robbed of endless eating, just do something else – liberate your nights. Learn to salsa. Play cribbage. Yodel. Embark on a journey through Dickens or Jilly Cooper. Go to bed. Demote eating and start to live.

✳ **And finally** . . . One more thing: eat supper at a reasonable time, leaving yourself at least a couple of hours to digest before you go to bed. That way, you'll sleep well and wake refreshed.

11 EAT MORE . . . OF THE RIGHT THINGS

Life shouldn't be an exercise in abstinence and purgatory. It should be fun and satisfying, and definitely full of food. What you need to know, though, is that everything works out fine just so long as you eat loads of some things and not a great deal of others. There's no mystifying formula to it, no secret recipe. We all know, deep down, what's good for us, even though the view may be momentarily obscured by a large portion of apple crumble and custard. Some foods are just more equal than others and we have to nail the nuts and bolts to have any hope of mastering the more challenging stuff to come. So, a few reminders. Try to:

✳ **Get complex**. Swap simple sugars for unrefined carbohydrates which keep you going for longer, like a Duracell bunny. Opt for carbs which are slow-burning (oats, brown basmati rice, stone-ground bread) rather than fast-burning (fudge cake, crumpets, anything by Mr Kipling). This is your best bet to bypass the sugar cycle – the crave-consume-crash-crave-consume-crash spiral which we all know so well. The short explanation of this pernicious loop is that highly refined carbs, by spiking your blood-sugar levels, encourage your pancreas to produce insulin. Insulin, for the purposes of this argument, is your demon, your nemesis within. It's a cunning opponent, too, with more than one weapon at its disposal. First, it reduces the level of glucose in the bloodstream by diverting it into various body tissues for immediate use – or by storing it as fat. It also inhibits the conversion of body fat *back* into glucose for the body to burn. So insulin has a double-pronged attack: it facilitates the accumulation of fat and then guards against its depletion. Insulin also acts on the brain to make you eat more and on your liver to manufacture more fat, and on the fat cells in your belly to store that fat. See? What a total fiend. A lovely steady blood-sugar level – as encouraged by those slow-burn carbs which take time and energy to digest – will stop your nervous system demanding that you stock up on fuel. In other words, eat them and you won't feel as hungry. How simple was that?

✴ **Eat more brown food**. 'People who eat white bread have no dreams!' proclaimed Diana Vreeland. If you have ever attempted to create an interesting sandwich using a white sliced loaf, you will see her point. The project is doomed from the get-go, even if you add chilli jam or interesting cured meats from Spain. Even the term 'white bread' has come to mean something bland and conventional, pappy and tasteless. Why would you want to eat that? Brown bread, by contrast, is well bred. If you haven't already, swap immediately. John Cusack, by the way, is said to avoid all white food – flour, sugar, rice, the lot. Most refined carbs are white, so it's a decent rule of thumb. If you can't commit to 100 per cent brown, try bread made with natural occurring 'albino' wholewheat, which looks white and acts brown (also known as 'white wheat', it doesn't have the tannins and phenolic acid found in the outer bran of red wheat, which some folk think give a bitter taste to wholewheat products).

✳ **Go for greens**. Yes, the old fruit-and-veg chestnut. But worth promoting – not just for the fibre and good vibes, but also because vitamin C, among its many health benefits, may well be crucial for weight management. According to researchers from Arizona State University, individuals who consume an adequate amount of vitamin C burn 30 per cent more fat during moderate exercise than those who don't get enough of the stuff. They also showed that too little vitamin C in the bloodstream correlates with increased body fat and waist measurements. So go to it, remembering that vitamin C is fragile and easily lost – so if you're cooking your vegetables, do it quickly and tenderly, as if pulling a splinter from a loved one's thumb.

✳ **Pick purple**. If you want to be truly in step with fashion (and Mariah Carey), go mauve. It will up your vitamin intake at a stroke. Beetroot, aubergines, blueberries, acai berries, plums, purple carrots, purple cauliflower, figs, olives, purple asparagus ... Foods of this colour are thought to be among the best natural sources of antioxidants and vital vits, and should be added to your menu along with greens. As Mariah herself says, 'I used to wake up and say, "What do I want to eat?" Now, rather than order any old thing that tastes good, I'll say, "What will keep me at the size where I feel better about myself?"' Borscht, that's what!

✳ **Find your pulse – learn to love the lentil**. Sadly, lentils have long had a bad press, ever since the hippies of the sixties appropriated them and based an entire philosophy on their simple, peaceful appeal. Lentils, together with other legumes, have been part of the human diet since Neolithic times, and with good reason. In the Bible, Esau was tricked into selling his birthright for a pottage of lentils (Genesis 25:34) – and, really, who could blame him? They are packed with protein, fibre, vitamin B and other absolute vitals such as iron and folic acid. Little legumes like the lentil, the chickpea and myriad varieties of dried bean, though unassuming on the shelf, are dynamite in the diet – in soups, in veggie burgers, in the glory that is tarka dahl – deftly balancing blood-sugar levels while providing that all-important steady, slow-burning energy.

What's more, there are so many lentils to try – brown ones, red ones, yellow ones and green ones. There are golden ones and black Beluga ones, and even a big yellow Mexican one called a Macachiados. My favourite, though, is the funky little Puy lentil, which does all the stuff your average lentil can do, but manages to be fashionable to boot.

✳ **Widen your repertoire to include grains you've not yet encountered**. Instead of relying on wheat – such a cliché – be wild and promiscuous in your grain consumption. Go for the wholesome whole ones, boasting way more micronutrients and fibre than their stripped-down cousins. In search of interesting slow-release-energy foods, try spelt, quinoa, bulgar and buckwheat. Too humdrum? Flirt with amaranth or teff. You'll find them in a health-food store, and you can chuck them in salads, soups and stews, or serve them as a jaunty side-dish to impress your friends. If that all seems like a bridge beyond, simply swap your refined white rice for brown rice. There are so many reasons to try, not least (whisper it) because brown rice *actually tastes of something*.

12 EAT MEALS, NOT SNACKS

In the past two decades, what we eat has changed beyond recognition. While much of it gives good reason to rejoice (California rolls! Mizuna leaves! Eleven different types of olive!), the evolution of our eating habits has meant we eat more. More food. More snacks. More of the time.

Not only are our servings bigger, with those cunning 'deep dish', 'big eat' and 'mega' deals out there to skittle us with their sheer licence-to-fill bulk, but also, between bucketfuls, our propensity for snacking is extraordinary. Today, there are very few stretches of time that remain food-free. A business meeting? Hey, have a muffin. Waiting for a train? Grab a cookie. Stopping for petrol? Don't forget the doughnut! Run your eye along the snack aisle at your local supermarket and be amazed by the breadth of choice out there. Scotch-egg bars. Teriyaki Kettle Chips. Giant Quality Street. The UK snack industry, though still in its infancy and lagging well behind the US, is worth around £9 billion a year, expanding all the while to service our new grazing, tableless lifestyles.

This snack-fest has changed the very shape of our days, with sociologists reporting that Americans have added to the traditional big three 'eating occasions' – breakfast, lunch and dinner – an as-yet-untitled fourth that lasts *all day long*. One study from Harvard found that Americans are not consuming any more calories at mealtimes than they did two decades ago, but they have almost doubled their consumption of calories from snacks and fizzy drinks between meals. And we Brits are not far behind.

These devilish bites are what the food industry calls 'ambient foods', designed for 'transient' consumers who crave 'instant grats'. Trendwatching.com, a company which monitors and labels these things, calls this our Snack Culture, noting, for example, that US sales of 100-calorie packs of crackers, chips, cookies and candy grew nearly 30 per cent in 2007. OK, petals, this may be low-cal. It may be novel, even cute. But is it food? At this point, it's worth noting a recent Dutch study which found that fun-size snack packs in fact encourage you to eat *more*, not less; participants who ate from 'guilt-free' mini packs ate more because they were not exercising the self-control demanded by a bigger bag. Here's more to digest:

✻ **The following things are not food, so don't put them in your mouth**: 'hand-held snacks', 'snacks on the go' and 'snack kits'. If you can pick it, dip it, pop it – do yourself a favour. Drop it. Similarly, if you have to unpeel three layers of advertising to get at the nosh, it's probably not worth the bother.

✻ **Try to eat at a table**. And no, as Michael Pollan rightly points out in his brilliant book *In Defence of Food*, your desk does not count. Today, for many, the concept of a 'family meal' – served at a table, with proper knives, forks and conversation, is as old-fashioned as the concept of darning socks or doing hospital corners. We have become a microwave- and freezer-based life-form. Introducing a table into the proceedings not only upgrades the whole experience; it makes you mind your food. This is good. Remember that only animals eat standing up. If forced, by dint of deadlines and the demands of your day, to eat lunch at your desk, surprise yourself with a change of plan. Instead of trooping up to Eat or Pret for one of those fat, wet sandwiches, go to that Italian deli or Spanish grocery on the corner. Buy a few slivers of prized ham, a handful of salty black olives, a vine of plum tomatoes and some bread for dipping into delicate green virgin oil. Let your screensaver gaze on in envy as you enjoy a proper little feast. Yes, it took longer to assemble and longer to eat, but you'll still remember it come home time.

'Americans have added to the traditional big three "eating" occasions – breakfast, lunch and dinner – an as-yet-untitled fourth that lasts *all day long*.'

✴ **Try not to eat alone**. Left to my own devices, and without the scrutinizing glare of my husband, I have been known to eat an entire family-sized pizza, starting at twelve o'clock and working my way clockwise all the way round to noon again. Alone, a human is like a hamster and will happily travel from one end of a packet of chocolate digestives to the other without pausing to blink. Eating in company, by contrast, serves to restrain speed, slovenliness and wanton behaviour (as one who has tried it, I can vouch for the fact that it is embarrassing to have thirds in front of guests). Do bear in mind, though, that eating with gluttonous belly-gods will almost certainly turn you into one too. If you have a large friend, invite them out for a jog, not round for a roast.

53

✱**Avoid enormous food**. I am constantly vexed by the pails of popcorn we're forced to buy at the movies. No one needs that much popcorn. Not ever. Not even to get through a Tom Cruise film. Broadly speaking, if the container is bigger than your head, don't buy it (you'll save yourself a fiver in the process). I am fond of the experiment performed by Professor Brian Wansink and his team at Cornell University which involved giving Chicago movie-goers tubs of five-day-old popcorn. Some got it in medium-sized buckets, others in large buckets. The leftovers were weighed at the end of the show – revealing that the people with the bigger buckets of stale popcorn ate 53 per cent more than the ones with smaller tubs. They ate it *because it was there*, which is pretty much why Mallory climbed Everest, but without the cardiovascular benefits. As the *New York Times* explains, 'People didn't eat the popcorn because they liked it. They were driven by hidden persuaders: the distraction of the movie, the sound of other people eating popcorn and the Pavlovian popcorn trigger that is activated when we step into a movie theater ...'

✱**Leave plenty of time**. If you're in a rush, you'll never make yourself a healthy sandwich or an interesting three-bean salad. You'll stop off at the petrol station and buy a chunky KitKat. You'll also be bound to 'inoculatte', which, according to the *Washington Post*, means 'to take coffee intravenously when you are running late'. Don't.

✱**Plan ahead and you'll cut back on snack attacks**. What will you eat tomorrow? What's for tea? Is there any of that guacamole left? Tune in to your fridge and your kitchen cupboards so that you can make informed decisions about your meals and make them sing. Don't just bump into food by accident. Don't graze on empty, fruitless snacks. Don't allow yourself to be ambushed by suppertime; it happens every day, give or take, so prepare the way. If you don't, that chicken-chow-mein delivery, that packet of HobNobs, that bag of Minstrels, will suck you in and spit you out on the wrong side of your new jeans, guaranteed.

13 OMIT NOTHING, FORBID NOTHING

This is not an endurance test, it is a life. So don't set yourself ridiculous targets. You will fail. Take your time and you will win.

Try a bit of self-help psychology when you're struggling with the temptation of that beckoning doughnut. Tell yourself you can have it. But you don't really need it. Not now, at any rate. You can have it later, if you still want it. By that point the craving may well have passed. Or you will have moved away from the bakery window and got on with your life . . .

If you simply can't resist, if the glinting sugar and the pudgy dough prove too much to bear, grant yourself an amnesty. But don't use an accidental collapse as a reason to binge until further notice, weeping as you ferry ice-cream into your face. It was a blip, not a felony. Rather than admonish yourself, rather than prohibit, you need to forgive, forget, move on. To Point 14, perhaps.

DETOX SCHMEETOX

You already know that you don't need to diet. What's more, if you eat a healthy, comprehensive and varied array of nutrients, you do not need to detox either. One of my favourite quotes on this topic comes from the Food Standards Agency's chief scientist Dr Andrew Wadge, who has urged people to ditch detox diets and supplements. On his FSA website blog, he writes, 'There's a lot of nonsense talked about "detoxing" and most people seem to forget that we are born with a built-in detox mechanism. It's called the liver. My advice would be to ditch the detox diets and supplements and buy yourself something nice with the money you've saved. Personally, I would recommend the new Neil Young and Steve Earle albums.' What you need, and a Neil Young album might well help, is to ditch dysfunction and discover a healthy balance that works for you.

14 COOK MORE

Let me introduce you to Marcie, a dear friend of mine. Marcie sleeps between Calvin Klein sheets, has exotic flora in Lalique vessels dotted around her Primrose Hill apartment, enjoys regular facials with someone called Aurora, boasts her own Pilates teacher, wears ridiculously expensive cashmere and uses Clinique's Moisture Surge Gel on her sensitive eye area. Her kitchen is, though she says it herself, impeccable, full of Wolf and Smeg and Gaggenau, all espresso machine, teppanyaki grill and brushed-aluminium wine cooler. Her empty dishwasher (always empty) smells of lemons. Her white bone-china is stacked in pleasing towers, waiting to be called up for duty. Marcie's impressive pull-out cupboards show off their contents to the laziest eye – whole nutmegs, aromatic cloves, a weird herb called Nigella, bought as a token of her affection for the nation's greatest cook. But get this. She never uses *any of it*. Not the cumin, nor the coriander seed. Not the dried dill, the oregano, the saffron stalks which look coquettish, like golden eyelashes. Marcie, though her kitchen screams gastronome, doesn't cook. She orders in. She eats out. But she doesn't cook. It reminds me of Jennifer Aniston's wonderful comment when she had just moved into her marital Malibu mansion with Brad all those years ago: 'Staying in is the new going out. It's nice to invite your friends over, have dinner parties, play poker. Not that I can cook, but I'm planning on learning and we have a great kitchen.'

We may not be as detached from the front line of cooking as Jen or Marcie, but many of us have developed a perverse relationship with our plates of late. In the UK, we spend £133 billion a year on food, but we chuck a third of it away. We devour TV chef shows, but have forgotten how to cook. Even if we're confident in the kitchen, able to pirouette between the béchamel sauce and the brulée torch with the assurance of a pro, who isn't too tired, too busy, too idle to pick up a potato peeler at the end of the day? As writer Zoe Williams says, 'We all know what to do with an aubergine but can't be arsed.'

If we want to lose weight, to eat well, perhaps we should be arsed. There is, after all, something so vital, so visceral, about cooking. I don't expect you to skin a rabbit or hang a pheasant. And as a working mother I recognize how very easy it is to let it slide – how tempting an Authentic Bistro chilled ready-meal can seem at the end of a hectic day. But stripped of its jazzy sleeve, what have you got? A beige lasagne made in a factory outside Purley? An anonymous savoury mush ladled from a steel vat by a bloke in a hairnet? Come on. Faced with the prospect of the chiller cabinet, it's important to think outside the box. Perhaps not always, but often. How hard is it for me to put a chicken in the oven, a squeeze of lemon and a rub of rock salt on its chest? To wash a lettuce? Make a dressing with Dijon, olive oil and sharp white-wine vinegar? Compared with ready-made meals, is there really a contest?

To really get a handle on your love handles, then, you need to get to grips with your food. Your dinner shouldn't say *ping*! It should say *mmm*. So follow Kelly Osbourne's advice and chuck out the microwave (ensuring no one is standing beneath your window first). Make a vow to develop a more intimate relationship with your food. Reconnect. 'Food!' we should think at the appropriate hour of the day. 'Brilliant!'

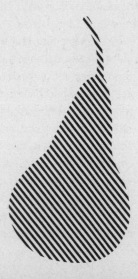

15 GO SLOW AND DIGEST YOUR FOOD PROPERLY

It seems a simple enough invocation, but just think about how much you bolt. Gulp. Rush. Janet Street-Porter's advice for a long and healthy life really ought to be emblazoned on your forehead in felt-tip pen: 'Eat as slowly as you can and never miss a meal' – increasingly important in a culture where everyone is always, always late. Just as Slow Food – the international movement opposing fast food and promoting dining as a source of pleasure – has taken hold in the collective consciousness, so Slow Eating ought now to settle in for the duration. By this I mean eating with intent. Eating to savour. History students among us may recall that witty aphorism, 'Nature will castigate those who don't masticate,' catchphrase of early diet guru Horace Fletcher – a fastidious fellow who promoted the idea that properly chewed food lessens the appetite, leading to weight loss and better health. Fletcher advocated chewing each mouthful thirty-two times – or until the food became liquid in the mouth – before swallowing. He even suggested that *liquids* be chewed to mix them properly with saliva. Henry James and John D. Rockefeller were both advocates, and probably made for quite dull dining companions as a result. But Fletcher was on to something: your mouth has a job to do in the breakdown of incoming morsels. Rush food through as if it's on a bullet train to nowhere and you are asking for trouble. So do chew a bit more. And don't gobble, guzzle, wolf or swig. Make a conscious effort to taste and enjoy your food. Put your knife and fork down between bites. Let your body know what's just hit it. Proper chewing is said to be the cheapest form of weight management, and if that doesn't sell it to you, nothing will.

While we're on the inside looking out, do try to get regular. I lived through the seventies, when every third person was on the F-Plan Diet, eating tons of bran buds in a bid to convey food from one end to the other without impediment. There's still, as ever, much to recommend fibre: it is found in the cell walls of plants –

in fruit, vegetables, wholegrains, cereals, nuts, seeds and beans – and is not digested when we eat. This means it is an ideal bulking agent, making us feel full sooner and staying in our stomachs longer than other food. It slows down our digestion rate – more lovely slow stuff – which means we stay full all the way from one roughage encounter to the next. It is well known, for instance, that wholegrain bread is twice as filling as the spongy white alternative. And, as an added bonus, fibre escorts fat through our digestive system, meaning that less of it is absorbed and lodged in the body. It is also a widely accepted, though little discussed fact that at any given moment a quarter of the population is suffering from constipation. Nix it by hydrating, walking and branning. Going slow is all very well in the kitchen, but not in the bathroom.

FAST FOOD:
HOW TO TELL IF YOU'RE SPEED FEEDING

✳ If you are talking with your mouth full, you're going too fast.

✳ If you get hiccups, you're going too fast.

✳ If you've already got to the end of this paragraph, you're going too fast.

✳ If you ask for the bill before you've finished the cheesecake, you're going too fast.

✳ Ditto if you spill things down your front . . .

✳ If you can't remember what you had for lunch . . .

✳ If you take a phone call during supper . . .

✳ If your lunch-hour lasts twelve minutes . . .

✳ If you have a favourite flavour of Rennie.

All of these things are signposts that you are eating too quickly, and you are unlikely to digest your meals efficiently. This is not only a problem for anyone who has to dine with you. It is a big issue for your poor afflicted innards, and it can have a deleterious effect on your weight.

16 GIVE FOOD YOUR UNDIVIDED ATTENTION

Don't read, watch TV, text, drive or juggle as you eat. That way, you'll know when you're full (at which point, STOP).

In Japan, it is apparently considered rude to eat and walk at the same time, but somehow in the West our paths are populated by pedestrians stuffing in a muffin en route to somewhere vital. I am forever amazed by the number of people who manage to eat on the run. Noodles with chopsticks. Whoppers with extra cheese. Pizza, ribs, burritos. All leaking on to the shared space of Sauchiehall Street or the Number 94 to Shepherd's Bush.

If you want to develop a healthy relationship with your calories, give them a little space. 'Eating and drinking aren't errands,' says the author of *The Fat Fallacy*. 'It's not what you do on the way to something else.' Correct. It's something you do when you're hungry (not fidgety, not sad, not over the moon, but hungry). Too many of us eat on auto-pilot, in a daze. One in five of us snacks when we're bored; most of us will eat until a TV programme ends; some of us don't even know what's on the fork.

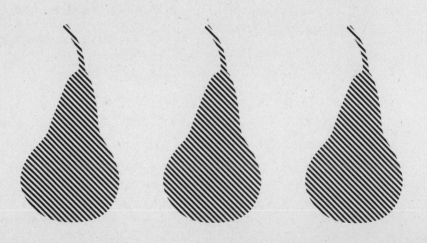

HOW NOT TO EAT:
YOU KNOW YOU'RE NOT ENGAGING WHEN . . .

* You find crumbs in your keyboard.
* The novel you're reading boasts thumb-prints of jam on page thirty-two.
* You have mastered eating while applying lipstick or (God forbid and forgive you) while you're on the loo.
* The person on the other end of the phone says, 'Are they salt & vinegar?'
* You've missed your stop.
* There's a Ben & Jerry's Chunky Monkey stain on your nightie (this is called a 'negligence' in our house).
* The sudoku is finished by dessert.
* You use three implements during supper: knife, fork and remote control.
* Your partner says, 'Do you want any more goulash?' and you say, 'What goulash?'
* You shift your gum to one side of your mouth to eat a croissant.

17 PLAY STRAIGHT – NO FOOD STASHES

I'm talking about the Galaxy bar in the fridge, the biscuits gently warping in your desk drawer, the Jelly Babies in the glove compartment. De-cache. De-stash. Dolly Mixtures under the bed? Eccles cake in your pocket? Stop hoarding food for future use. If you're the kind of person who ferrets food away, keep it on a shelf instead, like an ornament, not hidden behind a cushion on the sofa. Karl Lagerfeld, a man whom I adore despite his fantastic oddness, is said to keep 'red meat, alcohol and chocolate at home as a decorative accent to smell and see, but not eat'. Do *not* do this yourself unless you are already fantastically odd. Do, however, come clean. Be up-front, out and proud and rid yourself of guilty secrets.

Be aware (not obsessed, just aware) of what you eat on a daily, drudging, *whoa-did-I-really-eat-that-last-crumpet?* basis. In surveys, half of us admit to lying about how much we eat, and to eating in secret. All over the country there are women, lodged under the stairs or behind a convenient pot plant, cramming in the last of the fudge cake while backs are turned. I do it. You do it. One poll found that 50 per cent of women confess to having eaten an entire packet of biscuits in one go. There is, then, a below-radar food fest going on in kitchens, pantries and utility rooms throughout the land. If you're at it, notice it.

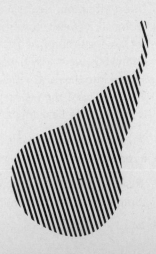

18 SURPRISE YOURSELF AND BREAK THE HABITS OF A LIFETIME

Studies reveal that up to 45 per cent of what we do every day is habitual – performed without thinking in the same location at the same time in the same dullard way. Think about the urge to check an email. To wipe a counter. To apply lotion. To grab a snack. It's why advertising works. It's why you trek through the supermarket each week on the same established route. 'Habits are formed when the memory associates specific actions with specific places or moods,' says Professor Wendy Wood of Duke University in North Carolina. 'If you regularly eat chips while sitting on the couch, after a while, seeing the couch will automatically prompt you to reach for the Doritos.' Now that we've hit Number Eighteen, it's high time to change the schedule. Get random, have chance encounters, leave room for manoeuvre and space for the unexpected. Fight the triggers of habit and you'll fight the fat.

'On a neurological level,' says psychologist Kerry Halliday, 'women plagued by weight issues need to develop positive pathways, not retread the negatives. It takes twenty-one days to break a habit – so, at first, every time you face a compulsion to eat too much, or to eat poorly, you need to face this head on. Try to install a behaviour that chips in to your established route. Go for a walk. Phone a friend. Get out of the house. Leave your desk. Divert attention, break thought patterns and change the picture.'

We all, however, possess a 'status quo bias', our quotidian lives set to a well-thumbed default position. We head for the same seat on the bus, we stay with the same TV channel as one programme segues into the next, we sheepishly follow the path of least hassle. What you need, then, is a series of minor movements. Small changes. No obsessions. Real differences. Stir it up, little darling, stir it up.

✷**Park as far away from the supermarket/work/the patisserie as possible**. That way – guess what? – you have to walk further.

✷**Be radical**. If you habitually eat in front of the TV or your computer screen, outlaw both. Commit to never again eating

63

in the office, at your desk or on the sofa. In a week or so, your habit – that regular, routine fodder-fest that you barely notice – will be reformed. Plus, you won't find toast crumbs in your keyboard or lodged down the back of the sofa.

✳ **Plot your pitfalls**. Note when your self-control is likely to crumble. If you're always starving when you get in from work, make sure there's a banana stashed in your bag to eat on the bus, so that you don't demolish a whole loaf as soon as you're through the front door. If you're prone to a late-night forage in the fridge, run a bath instead. Avoid the traps – that gormless peering into the fridge for inspiration, the welcoming grin of a bread bin stacked with doughy goodies, the evening wine bottle stationed so conveniently on the coffee table. If the kitchen is on your left, turn right. You may find yourself staring at a bookshelf instead, or on the patio talking to a neighbour about cherry blossom.

✳ **Don't plant yourself in a forest of calories and hope for the best**, for verily you will grow fat and complacent. Adjust your life to dodge your food fetishes. If you can't go into Starbucks without buying a blueberry muffin (380 calories), don't go into Starbucks. If you pick up a Bounty bar every time you buy a newspaper, have your newspaper delivered. Study the enemy and don't put yourself in the line of fire.

✳ **Have an idea of your own personal Habit Map** – the locations which, without fail, suck you in and spit you out again, having just cruised through a whole heap of superfluous food. My own map would go something like this (giving both the enemy's coordinates and weapon of choice):
M&S: Extremely Chocolatey Mini Bites.
Boots: roast chicken and stuffing sandwich, Cadbury's Snack Shortcake (six-pack).
Starbucks: Rise & Shine muffin and decaf double-tall cappuccino.
Pret à Manger: cinnamon Danish.
Carluccio's: almond croissant(s).
And so on, my entire day punctuated with excuses to stop off

and revisit an old favourite. Your mission, should you choose
to undertake it, is to break these habits. Take another route to
work. Walk on by. Shop elsewhere. Cross the road when you know
there's a food grenade in your path – an all-day breakfast, say, or
an espresso stall which does a quite brilliant pain au chocolat.

 Have a handle, too, on your Food Memory Map – the behaviour
around eating that stems from your background, your childhood,
the Proustian moments you may have stored in the dusty back-
rooms of your mind. It may not be madeleines. It may be KFC
or an entire brick of Dairy Milk. It may be lardy cake or pasties
or the Fondant Fancies your grandmother served on doilies in the
dappled mote-light of her front room. These atavistic delights are
sewn into your soul, right there in your deep-buried snake-brain,
and your reaction to them now, as a grown-up, is a potent one.
It's enough to have you reaching for an extra dumpling simply
because it makes you feel safe and loved and liberated from the
constraints and concerns of adulthood. Just be aware, that's all.

19 TACKLE TEMPTATION

Ah, we all know how easy it is to make soaring promises about
how little we'll eat tomorrow, how far we'll run next week. A
marathon in March! Crispbreads from Friday! It is considerably
more difficult to modify your present-tense behaviour – to get
off that couch, right now, before the ad break finishes – than to
plot your future brilliance. This is what social psychologists call
'dynamic inconsistency' – the gap between what you plan in good
faith and what you do in real time. The issue, as Richard Thaler and
Cass R. Sunstein demonstrated so deftly in their hit book *Nudge*,
is that humans respond to a given situation based on their state
of arousal, whether they are 'hot' or 'cold'. When in the cool,
disinterested state, we tend to underestimate the hotty effect

of arousal. It's all very well hatching plans to lose a stone utilizing the Just Say No principle – but when confronted with a bowl of fat chips, tempting, crisp and salty from the fryer, when faced with the prospect of a fascinating cheese board or a second bottle of that extremely good red ... well, resistance is suddenly futile.

'The food industry has spent a great deal of effort and money laying subtle traps to get our snouts in the trough.'

The problem is that everything around us – advertising, aromas, opinions – exerts a subtle pull on our behaviour and our salivary glands. The food industry, driven by profit, wants us to eat. All the time. And it has spent a great deal of effort and money laying subtle traps to get our snouts in the trough. We all know about the fresh-bread smells in supermarkets and how they lead you blindly to the till in the company of cinnamon waffles and a quart of double cream – but the psychological manipulation goes deeper by far. You're more likely to buy an iced bun in a shop which smells of coffee. People are known to order dessert in a restaurant simply because of the kind of music being played. We apparently spend more in a supermarket if we shop in an anti-clockwise direction ...

The best you can do is to plan ahead to resist the siren call from that fourth glass of Chardonnay, the special offer on Terry's Chocolate Oranges or that cold sausage in the fridge. Over the next nine chapters, you'll equip yourself with hundreds of ways to do just that. For now, simply recognize temptation for what it is. Temporal. Transient. Breathe, move on, it's gone. Feel strong. If a retail environment smells delicious, it's time to smell a rat. Oh, and shop backwards. Unleash your inner contrarian.

20 UNDERSTAND HUNGER

Many of us never give our bodies the chance to feel even the slightest bit empty, surfing as we do from one snack to the next. Research has found that most overweight people have completely lost the hunger sensation; eating has become their response to all emotion, no matter what they feel.

Do, then, try at least once a day to put off eating until you feel hungry. Not ravenous, but more than just peckish. Real physical hunger, rather than a mild longing for lunch. Give your stomach the chance to growl at the postman – but don't, please, abstain utterly from food and drive yourself insane with craving. Here's why: scientists have found that ghrelin, a hormone produced in the stomach which signals hunger to the brain, can make *all* food desirable. This may once have provided an adaptive advantage to humans, who needed to feast on any amount of garbage when times were lean. But now? Calamitous.

According to a report in the journal *Cell Metabolism*, the hormone stimulates the same reward centres of the brain that have been linked to drug-seeking behaviour. Aha. This explains so much human endeavour. The meat-pie business . . . Hot dogs . . . Squirty cream . . . Mr Whippy . . . Why a bucket of divine, delicious, delectable fried chicken seems so appalling once you've demolished half of it and appeased the ghrelin gremlin. As actress Beth McCollister puts it, 'Food is like sex: when you abstain, even the worst stuff begins to look good.' Knowing this, you need to get a handle on your hunger, noticing it but keeping it comfortably at bay. Recognize what hunger feels like, so you can distinguish between real hunger and other reasons for wanting to eat. But don't let your hunger take over completely, or you may be driven to binge on anything that isn't nailed to the floor.

21 DRINK MORE WATER

It is an established tenet of dieting folklore that water will somehow miraculously facilitate weight-loss – as if it gushes through your system seeking out fat cells as it goes, transporting them south like logs over the Niagara Falls. Alas, this is not the case.

There is, however, evidence to suggest that increasing water consumption will speed up your metabolic rate (the rate at which calories are burned). A study from Berlin's Franz-Volhard Clinical Research Centre found that subjects increased their metabolic rate by 30 per cent after drinking about 17 ounces of water. Increasing water consumption by 1.5 litres a day would burn an estimated additional 17,400 calories over the course of a year, equating to a weight loss of around five pounds. American researchers have concluded that while there's no scientific reason to drink the 'recommended' eight half-pint glasses of water a day, up to 75 per cent of us *are* chronically dehydrated (a dry mouth, incidentally, is the last sign of dehydration, not the first).

There are other watertight reasons for drinking more fluids. Water fills your belly, for one, which is why so many people swear by drinking a glassful before each meal. It also stops you mistaking thirst for hunger (37 per cent of people are thought to have a thirst mechanism so weak that they misinterpret thirst as hunger). Drinking water keeps your mouth occupied when it would otherwise be anticipating a crafty doughnut. It's a natural appetite suppressant, and, though it won't wash fat cells away, it will flush out salts and toxins and other superfluous junk your body could do without. What's more, the University of Washington has shown that one simple glass of water before bed shuts down midnight hunger pangs for 100 per cent of dieters. That's some hit rate, and all for nowt.

BILGE WATER: WHY TAP IS TOP

In Britain we spend an annual £2 billion a year on bottled water, a product which boasts one of the highest mark-ups in the known universe. Thanks to a gradual raising of eco-consciousness, however, ordering tap water is increasingly fashionable, and a good thing too: in the UK, at least 99 per cent of tap water passes quality sampling, and costs up to ten thousand times less than bottled. For the finest taste, filter it and keep it in an earthenware or glass vessel in the fridge . . .

Some of us, of course, still cherish the sass and security of the water bottle – its ease of availability, its portability, the subtle little signals it gives out. If tap water really doesn't float your boat, find a water that you do like; that way, you'll drink more of it. Personally, I have always been partial to Badoit and San Pellegrino because they have small, well-behaved bubbles and a mineral content which appeals to me. Jennifer Aniston is said to prefer Fiji water, a rich source of silica (accounting, one would like to think, for her swishy hair and glowing skin). If you dine at Claridges, you'll be offered a Water Menu, featuring the superior 420 Volcanic for £50 a litre – though you can, if you are both stingy and sensible, order a jug of 'London water' free of charge.

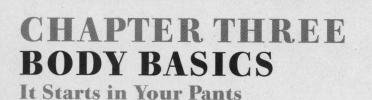

CHAPTER THREE
BODY BASICS
It Starts in Your Pants

With those first principles stashed under our belt, it's time to get down to the bottom line. A lack of body confidence means that we tend to cover everything up, hoping a great swathe of fabric will camouflage us and disguise our wobbles and worries in a crowd. It won't. It will make us look like a marquee.

A great body shape, in common with a great building, starts with reliable foundations. Your weight does not exist in limbo, some notional number that defines your very essence. Your weight is your whole body – all of it, from fingertips to eyelashes, and not just those love handles and hateful extra pounds that are getting you down. So you need to begin to nurture a positive vision of a whole new you. Think it, see it and pretty soon you'll be it. Start at the ground floor and work your way up.

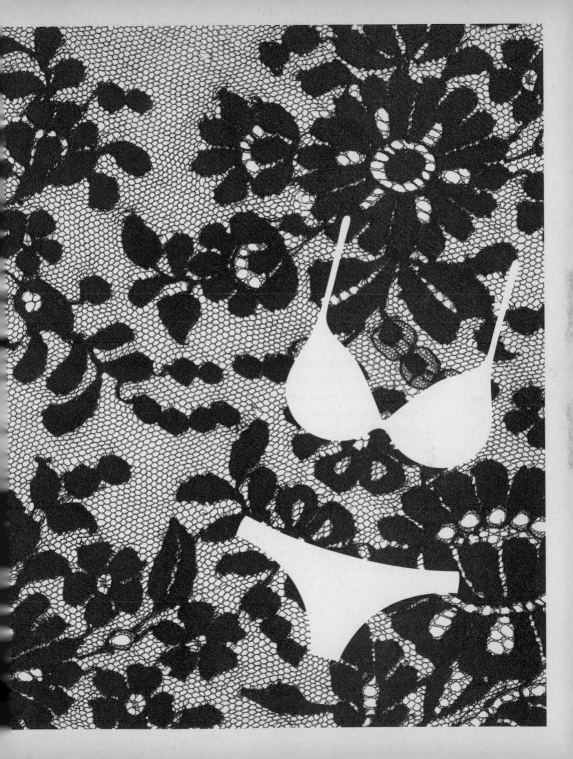

22 PERFECT YOUR POSTURE

We're in the business of looking willowy, right? Lean? We're aiming to look less breeze-block, more long-tall-drink-of-water. Now think about an orang-utan. Lovely creature, yes. Willowy, no. Giraffes are willowy. You do not want to look as though your knuckles trail the floor when you walk. You want to give the impression that you could reach the highest leaves on the tallest tree, and this applies just as well to five-foot-nothings as it does to six-foot-somethings. The difference is all in your posture.

Interestingly, it is often tall women who have the worst posture, perhaps because they are self-conscious about their height. Others are embarrassed by their breasts, seeking to minimize them by hunching the shoulders and rounding the lower back. As a result, we end up with a concertina tummy and a mild stoop, which does nothing at all for a cashmere sweater.

Good posture has all manner of beneficial effects. It means your skeleton is aligned, with your bones in the right place and not under untoward stress. It also makes you look way better in a cocktail dress. So hold your head up high (which also helps with the double chin), pull those abs in, raise the rib-cage, lengthen that neck and away you go.

Clothes, incidentally, can have a significant effect on posture. A tight-fitting jacket and good shoes can change the way you stand and walk. If you have ever trolled along like Bilbo Baggins because you're wearing flip-flops, if you have ever stretched like a kitten in mohair, if you've ever walked like a boss in a trouser suit, you'll recognize the truth in these words.

TA-DA! DO THE MOUNTAIN POSE

So you want to walk tall? Instead of parading up and downstairs with an encyclopedia balanced on your head, as advocated by Swiss finishing schools, try yoga. The practice is one of the best routes to flexibility, body consciousness and refined posture. If your day is just too manic to allow a proper session, simply doing Mountain Pose, known in Sanskrit as Tadasana, for five minutes each morning can have a profound influence on your physical and mental well-being and improve your posture no end. Here's how:

* Feet hip-width apart.

* Toes spread.

* Weight evenly distributed between feet.

* Stand tall.

* Draw shoulders back and down.

* Tuck tailbone under.

* Chin parallel to floor.

* Hands hang at sides.

* Relax. Breathe. Be still.

* Yoga manuals tend to say things like 'Allow your head to float upwards off your shoulders,' which is clearly barking. But *do* try to clear your mind – it may be your only chance in this crazy day to do so. Stop thinking about what you're having for supper. Yes, the windows really do need a clean. But this is your time. Be here now.

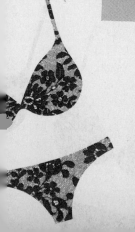

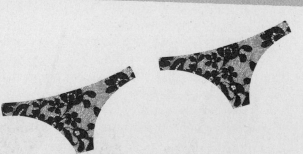

23   GET FITTED FOR A NEW BRA

As Kate Winslet says, 'I start with the bra. If the bra's right, everything else falls into place.' Don't you adore that? So utterly effortless that it makes you want to lie down on a couch and eat fudge. But Ms Winslet is on to something. The right bra – by which I mean one that not only rises to the occasion (whether that's putting out the bins or dancing till dawn), but one which *fits* – is a diet dream.

A properly fitted bra will treat your entire body to an instant upgrade. It will improve your posture (see above), streamline your silhouette, separate your bosom from your waist, draw the eye away from your tum and fool onlookers into thinking you've lost half a stone or half a decade. It could well be the best thirty quid you'll ever spend.

The issue, though, is that so few of us *are* wearing the right bra. A full 86 per cent of British women are thought to be wearing the wrong one right now, and I'll bet my Poupie Cadolle Plunge Petale Double Net Brassière with Frou Frou Trim that you're one of them. Breasts are brilliant – ask anyone – and yet we routinely house them in a garment that amounts to little more than an afterthought, as if we're stashing them there for safe-keeping until they might come in useful. Are you perhaps ladled into a cup too small, so that you threaten to spill over like a tremulous soufflé? Do you have four breasts courtesy of a badly fitted bra? Do you identify with P. G. Wodehouse's description: 'She looked as if she had been poured into her clothes and had forgotten to say "when"'?

If so, it's time to get to grips with your tits. I did this myself not long ago, by visiting the renowned rooms of Rigby & Peller in Conduit Street, home of all that is fitting in brassières and purveyor of undergarments to the Queen. Her Maj gazes down from a photograph behind the till, superbly contained in full Rigby rigging and royal regalia, her chest somehow staunch and dependable, the very manifestation of the British monarchy. I arrived a size 36C, and, after a rather intimate moment in a cubicle with a delightful woman named Gina, I emerged a 30E. I was astonished. You could have knocked me over with a marabou mule. And it all happened in a flash. Gina took one look at my naked back and knew that I had been roaming the land for decades saddled with the wrong tack. Within seconds I was eased into a bra that was both substantially bigger (in the cup) and substantially smaller (in the band) than I had been wearing for donkey's. This, it transpires, is the classic error and one which is simplicity itself to fix. The result? Things were certainly looking up. I'd gone from dugs to jugs, from droop to boop – and all because the bra was doing the work. I strolled out on to New Bond Street and a builder shouted 'Great bangers!' at me from his scaffold. I would have tossed an 'Oafish git' in his direction if I hadn't been quite so busy feeling pleased with myself.

And so my new breasts and I have been out and about, meeting and greeting. My husband is delighted with this turn of events, and has taken to buying me a new wardrobe of bras to cope with this sylphic Barbie to whom, it turns out, he is married. So, all in all, everyone's a winner.

Interestingly, over the past decade alone, the average UK bra size has increased from 34B to 36C/D, with almost a third of British women currently wearing a D cup or above; more D+ cups are sold in the UK than anywhere else in Europe. If your own cup runneth over, go to Bravissimo, which caters expressly for what they call 'big-boobed women'. Either way, it's well worth going to a professional to be fitted; high-street stores tend to give you a cursory once-over and a flick of a tape measure, sending you off to the till with the word 'average' stamped on your forehead. Specialists like Gina are, by contrast, trained in the art of the bra, and you'll be surprised how far off-target your current effort is. According to Rigby & Peller, we ought to be fitted every time we buy a bra. Changing hormone levels, the Pill, your diet and weight changes will all affect your bust size; it will almost certainly fluctuate, even in the relatively short term, so best keep abreast of your chest.

BRA BRILLIANCE IN A NUTSHELL

❋ Bras, like men, lose their potency over time, so get fitted for a new bra every six months, treating it like a trip to the dentist (but cheaper and way more fun).

❋ Take your time choosing a bra. Why hurry? This is worth three months in the gym. Or cabbage soup for six weeks.

❋ Once you and a professional have alighted on the correct size, lean forward into the bra.

❋ Run two fingers between breast and cup to ease everything into position.

❋ Adjust the straps – you want them firm but friendly.

❋ If the back band rides up, your bra is too big.

❋ Buy a bra which feels snug on its loosest hook setting: it will give with every wash.

❋ Your breast should completely fill the cup, but not overspill.

❋ If you have quad-boobs, your cup is too small.

❋ Larger cup sizes need underwiring for added support; an underwire should lie flat to the breast bone.

❋ Raise your arms. Your bra should stay put.

❋ If a bra fits well, it shouldn't pinch or poke or hassle you at parties.

❋ Check your bra by standing up straight – the centre of your bust should fall halfway between your elbow and shoulder. If it's gone south, you need to hoick it all back up.

❋ If you require assistance in the oomf stakes, technology has recently stepped right up: try Fashion First Aid's range of Boostits, Liftits, Concealits and Tapeits – a series of clever inserts which will perk up your chest, keep it under control or conceal pushy nipples. As an added bonus, once removed and rolled around in the palm of the hand, a Boostit apparently makes a very satisfying stress ball.

24 RECOGNIZE THE IMPORTANCE OF PANTS

Gosh, don't you just know when you've got it wrong? Who hasn't experienced the pestilential discomfort of the wedgie – that impish slice of thong lodged between cheeks, insinuating itself as you saunter down the street? You wiggle. You do a little two-step. You launch into the Charleston, but to no avail. Eventually – oh rats – you just *have* to stop and pluck it out, hoping that bystanders won't notice that you're fishing about up your jacksy.

Or how about those knickers with the elastic just a *smidge* too tight, the ones that leave a welt of smarting red across your belly, and your thighs in danger of losing their blood supply? Or the ones where the elastic has given up entirely, so that you are oddly vulnerable if running for a bus ... the ones where there's way too much going on and your silhouette has to cope with ribbons, ruffles, furbelows, lacing, trapdoors, pockets and witty one-liners scrawled across your bum ... the ones which clutch at your buttocks in too intimate a manner, as if testing for ripeness, leaving you with a vicious case VPL. Nothing, incidentally, adds pounds like VPL.

Of course, no twenty-first-century woman should suffer in this way; the advent of proper underwear ought to have wiped it out at about the same time that smallpox disappeared from the world stage. But still, there are so many ways to get your knickers in a twist. Few items in your wardrobe have such a huge impact – not only on your shape and your look, but also on your day. The wrong pants can put you off your game, lose you a tennis match, make you snap at your partner, prohibit potentially delightful sexual encounters and generally be ruinous to your well-being.

As you may surmise, I have spent the best part of a career charting the ups and downs of the nation's knickers. I lived – on behalf of *you*, dear reader – through the startling goosing of the 'body' in the eighties, the aggressive G of the nineties, the roomy succour of maternity pants, built to house a family of four and still leave room for a chocolate éclair. I have done big bloomers and tiny tangas, I've gone frou-frou, sporty, commando. And what I have learned from this odyssey can be distilled into a quartet of Pants Regulations which you'd do well to heed.

✳ **A thong is a glorious thing**. It is nearly not a knicker at all, more the *idea* of a knicker, making it the ideal partner for all manner of trousers, particularly those clingy ones which demand that your underwear should take a back-seat. G-strings may be less fashionable than in their heyday (when Alexander McQueen invented bumster trousers and we all, in a fit of collective hysteria, decided the crack was immensely cool), but you still need a handful in your arsenal to triumph in very demanding clothes.

✳ **Boy shorts will do the rest**. The cut is gracious to the lower curve of a bottom, which means it does the job of a G-string without the discomfort and with a trifle more decorum.

✳ **Fancy pants are great on a date**, but not a whole lot of good if you're looking for a smooth, lean line. They are, however, a superior short-cut to improving mood and body image (see below).

✳ **Sloggi**. It's the whole seamlessness that makes them work. They feel like a treat too – not a saucy, *ooh-la-la* treat, but a private, practical one. Seamless pants are ideal beneath unforgiving trousers – anything in white, anything with a high waist, anything with a jersey cling. My favourite seam-frees are called Commando, which just about says it all.

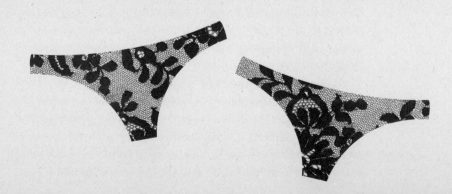

25 SHIFT YOUR SHAPE WITH SOLUTION LINGERIE

If you want to create the illusion of a flawless silhouette (Pah! Who doesn't?), you really need to put your underwear to work. Next time you're off out, do a little dance in front of the mirror. If you're all wobble and jiggle where you'd like to be taut and toned, get with the programme and invest in these mighty beasts. Don't, though, be dismayed when you unroll your new 'shape-wear'. This is not about sex, it's about shape. I suggest that you introduce yourself in private. You'll be confronted with a salami-skin of Lycra which promises to smooth your groove and send you out into the waiting world with a figure to make grown men whimper.

What's odd is that these pants are *massive*. Both in size and in popularity. It all started a decade or more ago on the red carpet, when stars were poured into foundation garments by their canny stylists, who well knew the insatiable curiosity of the paparazzi lens. Soon, we were all at it. Hey, if Jessica Alba, Carmen Electra and Halle Berry did it, we thought, then why not us?

Along came Spanx (revolutionary control-top pantyhose designed to contain all your wibbly bits – slogan: 'Don't worry, we've got your butt covered!') and a revolution ensued. They are, I'm reliably told, the undergarment of choice for Diane Sawyer, Hillary Clinton, Susan Sarandon and Joan Rivers. Renée Zellweger apparently 'flipped out over them' when they first appeared in 2000 and Oprah Winfrey still rarely takes hers off. Why? These über-pants, which, in certain formats, stretch from knee to bust, really do contain you like no other. Cleverly, they manage this feat of engineering without the excess blubber escaping at some other inopportune point (at the wrist, say).

These garments appeal not only because they do the business, but also, I suspect, because they are a million miles from the sturdy panty girdles you may have seen your grandmother roll on, a sight that probably stayed with you long after she was gone. My own grandmother would take hours to hoist and chivvy herself into position within the confines of a rubberized foundation garment, assisted by a liberal dusting of talcum powder and a very forgiving husband.

My, how times have changed. I wore a pair of these power pants just this morning, and I can tell you, they're a whizz at making you look lithe and lovely as you go about your daily business. You wouldn't want to wear them if you were in line for a saucy rendezvous, mind. But for times when it's all look and no touch? No contest.

THE **WHAT** AND **WHERE** OF SHAPE-WEAR

The issue today certainly isn't a lack of options. If anything, it's the sheer wealth of stealth-wear out there that can confuse a girl, as if a simple stroll around the lingerie department at your local store has turned into an all-out battle of the bulge. You can, should you wish, purchase a Hi-Waist Thigh Trimmer, a Deep-Plunge Body Suit, a Sculpted Bottom Boy-leg . . . or perhaps a super smoother, a waist cincher, a body briefer, a tummy tamer, and, yes, good old magic pants.

These days, it's all about technology. There's money in them there hills, which means that there is an awful lot of research and development going on behind the scenes, producing ever more effective under-things to spoon you out of bed and into the glare of the day. Very soon, we should be able to slap on a Super-Slimmer and disappear almost entirely, leaving our date to pick up the tab.

One reason for the runaway success of Solution Lingerie is that it allows women to wear all manner of fashion, no matter how revealing or advisable. If you're plunging at the front and back, splitting to the thigh and shearing to the tush, there's not a whole lot of places for a body to hide. Today, there is bound to be a shape-shifter just for you. Some will make you look like Ethel Merman; others more like Lance Armstrong. You'll just have to suck it in and see. Your only task in all of this is to ascertain precisely where your body needs most help, and then buy accordingly. As a rule, it's best to purchase in person rather than online; these things need a body to bring them to life. If you really can't get to your nearest department store for a comprehensive trying-on session, go to figleaves.com, a great website which stocks Spanx, Flexees, Rago, Body Wraps, the lot.

You'll notice that the latest innovations take inspiration from plastic-surgery techniques, using differing weights, stretch and strength of knitted elastic to echo the scalpel-cuts a surgeon might make to flatten the stomach, smooth the thighs or lift the buttocks. The upshot is an intelligent foundation garment, one which knows where to hold tight and where to relax, where to redistribute excess and where to let it loose – which scores the wearer a little more comfort and a good deal more confidence when exiting a taxi. Unsurprisingly, the company that specializes in just such a product (Dr Rey) sold $1.5 million worth of shapewear in its first weekend of trading.

My personal favourite, given my own soft spots, is the Yummie Tummie – a series of tanks and tees designed by Heather Thomson, a fashion associate of Beyoncé Knowles and Jennifer Lopez. The tops, available on yummietummie.com, feature a secret mid-section which holds in a belly and minimizes muffin top. 'The effects of Yummie Tummie are dramatic for the wearer, both physically and mentally,' says Thomson. Well, alleluia! Ideal for a woman like me who would gladly sell her belly on eBay, or swap it for an interesting set of spoons.

Whatever you choose – the 'skincarewear', perhaps, or the strapless body reducer – you're bound to shave off a good few pounds, and all for the cost of a new pair of shoes. You'd be a fool not to. As if to clinch the deal, we're now starting to see the arrival of shape-wear for men. The *Wall Street Journal* has reported on the burgeoning market for 'support boxers' to lift and firm the backside and 'waist eliminators' to tame the gut. If your man's in a mirdle, then surely you should be too?

26 LEARN HOW TO WALK WELL

As dear, dear Larry Olivier once declared, 'Give me the shoes and I've got the part!' Heaven knows, some of us need all the help we can get. I hate to carp, but British women seem peculiarly afflicted with poor gait, our feet slapping on the moist pavement as if there's bound to be bad news just around the corner. Worse, just watch most British brides as they galumph down the aisle in their thousand-pound frocks and dainty satin mules. My friend Josephine walked to the altar like the front half of a shire horse, which rather ruined her Vera Wang.

Mastering the gentle art of walking is a simple fix which can make weight appear to fall from a hunched and folded frame. I recommend walking lessons to anyone who has ever fallen downstairs into a party of new work colleagues gathered in a basement bar (me), anyone who has fallen *upstairs* while carrying a mug of hot chocolate (me) and anyone who regularly wears odd shoes (not odd as in 'unmatching', but odd as in 'inappropriate' – again, me).

Here is a tip-top lesson in how to walk gracefully. The marvellous Jean Broke-Smith (former principal of Lucie Clayton's etiquette school) would tell you to stand up tall, clench your derrière, and move forward with your heels following a line along the floor, and your toes pointed out just a bit. First place one foot in front of the other, then gracefully transfer your weight on to the heel of the front foot, then through the foot and on to the toe, as you pick up the back foot, place it in front, and so on. The idea is that you glide, with poise and balance, and with, I'm told, Jean's voice chanting 'heel-instep-toe, heel-instep-toe' in your head.

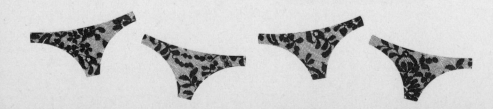

HOT TO TROT:
HOW TO WALK LIKE A SUPERMODEL

Though you still see the occasional pantomime horse, most models know how to walk well, a talent honed through years of practice. As model Jessica Stam says, 'First impressions are a big deal, whether you're walking up to the podium to give a presentation or into a restaurant for a blind date ... When a woman walks more confidently, it can really affect the way other people see her – and the way she feels about herself.' If you've ever watched Naomi Campbell's sashay or Gisele Bundchen's confident stomp, you'll know what Stam is getting at. Here's how to do it their way, for those days when you want to take a room by storm:

* Shoulders back and down, head straight, chin up, eyes focused gently at middle distance.

* Pelvis forward a little. Not too much or you will topple over backwards and land in a lap.

* Rather than glide in the Lucie Clayton way, place the *ball* of your foot down first, not the heel. Think Margot Fonteyn.

* Toes face forward. One foot is placed in line with the next, so your footprints would make a straight line in the sand. You are not a duck, so don't waddle.

* Take longish strides, raising your whole foot off the ground as you go.

* Engage your abs to stabilize yourself, then relax at the hip. That way, you'll manage all manner of frivolous shoes like a pro.

27 BUY A CORSET

In my hometown of Brighton, down a suitably Dickensian alley, is the She Said Erotic Boutique, a crooked little shop, home to a fetching collection of ostrich feathers and marabou, silken brassières and cheeky pants. The shop assistants all have hand-span waists, wild-cherry lips and cute, choppy fringes, true mistresses of the burlesque and dab hands at making a woman – any woman – come over all drop-dead femme fatale. One visit and you're guaranteed to drop a dress size, simply by discovering the incomparable power of stays. Victoria Beckham has known this since stage school. Kylie too. And Dita. So what's keeping you?

I went to She Said recently and bought a corset, a golden satin number with black lace trim and eight wicked suspender straps. It was called the 'Moulin Rouge', cost £170, and once I'd been chivvied into it, there I was: all bosom, all curves, all twenty-two inches of waist. After years of griping about the abomination of corsetry and any other contraption that turns women into dolls and men into dogs, it was here that I had my Damascene conversion. I was Madame Pompadour, Nell Gwynne, Scarlett Johansson on a flight of scarlet stairs ... An hourglass figure, I told my reflection in the mirror, is just sensational. It graces a body with curves and swoops, and spoons a chest into position like a couple of vanilla pies. Who would willingly turn that down?

The flirtatious play-off between enhanced bosom, contained tummy and diminished waist is of course pure female, a truth recognized throughout history. Consider the iconic images of womankind, and the waist almost always plays a starring role. *The Rokeby Venus* by Velázquez, *The Swing* by Fragonard, Scarlett O'Hara clutching the bedpost as she's drawn into her stays, Dior's New Look, Monroe, Mansfield, Madonna ... The picture is constant: an erotic conflation of billowing skirts and minuscule, embrace-me waist.

According to our long-established socio-cultural norms, women ought to nip in at the equator. Indeed, at the *fin de siècle*, a girl's eligibility was judged by the size of her waist – which should be 'twice the circumference of her neck, which, in turn, should be twice the circumference of her wrist', as defined by the dressmakers' guidelines of the day. If you were to ask a social anthropologist, they'd explain that the imagery is so consistent because there is an evolutionary imperative at play. The 'magic ratio' of waist to hips is, for women, 7:10. 'That silhouette is going to have a sexual appeal at a primeval level,' argued Desmond Morris long ago. 'It's signalling the child-bearing pelvic girdle, there's no great mystery about that.'

'One visit and you're guaranteed to drop a dress size, simply by discovering the incomparable power of stays.'

Though we are, as a gender, tending towards a thickening of the waist over time, there is no reason I can see why you shouldn't enhance your assets with a little artifice. You can buy a corset in several types of retail outlet, of course, but I would advise you to go to a specialist corsetière (Google will direct you to your nearest) – if only for the thrilling experience of being laced into this peculiar contraption by a proper professional with a choppy fringe. You won't want to wear it to trolley around the supermarket or pick up the kids from school. But for those big, razzle-dazzle moments in a girl's life, nothing can quite match it. Wear your corset under your clothes, a clandestine thrill, or out and proud over a sleek shirt. Either way, it will snatch several pounds too and stow them somewhere unknown, out of reach.

28 KNOW THE POWER OF BLACK OPAQUE TIGHTS

Opaque tights are truly a gift from heaven. They are central to existence, one of the ten vital inventions since the dawn of time (the others are Superglue, Marmite, Tweezerman, stock cubes, Maybelline mascara, fire, wheels, ear plugs and Manolo Blahnik). Back in the eighties, when my young legs were rarely out of them, opaques possessed the indefinable talent of making your shins, ankles, calves and knees look slimmer. They did this without the need for dieting or scandalously priced body-buffing creams. They did it without fuss, without nudging you in the ribs and saying, 'Oi, you have *got to* check this out!' They just did it as a matter of course, nonchalantly, as if clothes performed this kind of miracle all the time.

'Opaque tights, like cowboy boots, are trapped forever in the revolving door of fashion – sometimes emerging on the cool side.'

On top of this, opaque tights concealed a comprehensive catalogue of sins, from knobbly knees to in-grown hairs, from cracked heels to pasty legs, from scraped shins to unintentional exposure of that bit on the back of your upper thigh which you never ever get to see yourself unless you are very committed to yoga. What's more, opaque tights were warm! They were comfortable! They came in all manner of deniers – and the thick ones lasted for months as long as you bought them from Wolford. What more could you want?

Well, not much – apart from the promise that these wonder-hose should be in fashion *always*. Sadly, this was not to be. Opaque tights, like cowboy boots, are trapped forever in the revolving door of fashion – sometimes emerging on the cool side to strut about, making a miniskirt look like dynamite and you look like one of Robert Palmer's guitar girls from the 'Addicted To Love' video. And then, just as you're feeling confident that your legs will never again look so W-O-W, opaques swing round to the other side, cast off and blackballed by all but the most diehard sartorial klutz.

The replacement, generally, is patterned tights, which, by some fascinating precept of style, manage to have precisely the opposite effect. I have never met a woman (or a man, come to that) whose legs are enhanced by fussy hosiery. Fishnets, yes. In fact, fishnets, fabulous. Seamed stockings? Of course. (Few optical tricks will elongate a leg like a tramline heading north.) But on no account should we indulge in marrow-coloured tights, unless we are playing Peter Pan. No Pucci swirls, no rococo curlicues, no witty squiggles. Chevrons, spots, lace and rainbow hoops should similarly be reserved for the under-fives, and even then I'd err on the side of caution. Instead, I suggest we all wear black opaques, regularly, persistently, as often as we wear jeans, often enough for people to notice and think, 'Hey, would you look at that? Opaques are back! It's fine to continue wearing mine.' This, my friends, is fashion democracy in action.

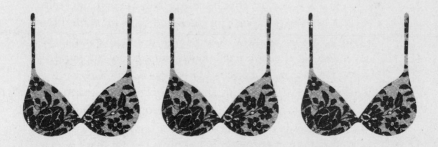

29 PUT ON YOUR BEST UNDERWEAR

I know women who have an entire collection of lingerie which they are 'saving for best'. These superb frillies lie in state, in a dark drawer or on a distant shelf, in tissue wrap or muslin bag, while the everyday drones of the underwear drawer – those tangas, briefs and bras in much-washed cotton – go about their duties. The posh stuff comes out to play only once in a very long while, on high days and holidays and evenings when there's the genuine prospect that they'll see action – from a lover, perhaps, or a competitive friend.

Admit it. When was the last time you wore that balconette bra in golden satin? The adorable set in coffee-coloured lace? The sugar-pink cami-knickers with the mocha ribbon lacing? Though we're buying ever more of the stuff, most of the time – because we're in a rush or in a rut – we don't wear gossamer panties and woo-hoo bras. We stick instead to what we know best. This generally boils down to routine stock in the greige colour range, worn in the earnest hope that we won't be knocked down by a bus or picked up by a stranger or find ourselves in a position where suddenly we have to show our knickers in public (getting changed at a spa, say, or falling off a bucking bronco at a barn dance). I was at school sports day just this week, and found myself jumping up and down as my son came fourth in the sack race. 'Nice panties,' my great friend Lou whispered in my ear. And thank heavens it was Lou, for these panties were not nice. They were as old as the hills and might even have once had the word 'Wednesday' printed on the front, though it had long since evaporated in the wash. It's possible I wore these pants to sit my finals, or my driving test, or on the lap of a man called Keith whom I might have married if only he hadn't been called Keith. A good twenty years down the line, and the pants are still desperately clinging to life, cheering my boy on as he jumps through the heat of a summer's afternoon.

So, I well understand the reasons for playing safe. Old pants are comfy pants. Reliable. My friend Nicky swears by several pairs which boast more than the regulation three holes, arguing that they have been with her through thick and thin and feel like dear old friends. Besides, silk knickers require special washing procedures. And leopard-print ruche-front bras can feel a trifle tarty for a nine a.m. breakfast meeting with the accounts department. BUT . . . there is nothing quite so delightful, so indulgent as wearing a flimsy, vulnerable nothing in whispering satin, a silk flower budding at the cleavage. Though I don't expect you to get dolled up like a box of truffles every single day, it is worth rolling out the tease on a fairly regular basis. Why? Psychology, stupid. If you treat yourself, you'll love yourself. You'll feel good about you, at an intimate, personal, mildly saucy level. Dressing as though you're expecting rain will influence the mood of your day. Dress like a goddess – even underneath that workaday navy trouser suit – and you just see what it does for your self-image. You may even find yourself having more sex. This, needless to say, is ace (see Point 86).

'Admit it. When was the last time you wore that balconette bra in golden satin? The adorable set in coffee-coloured lace? The sugar-pink cami-knickers with the mocha ribbon lacing?'

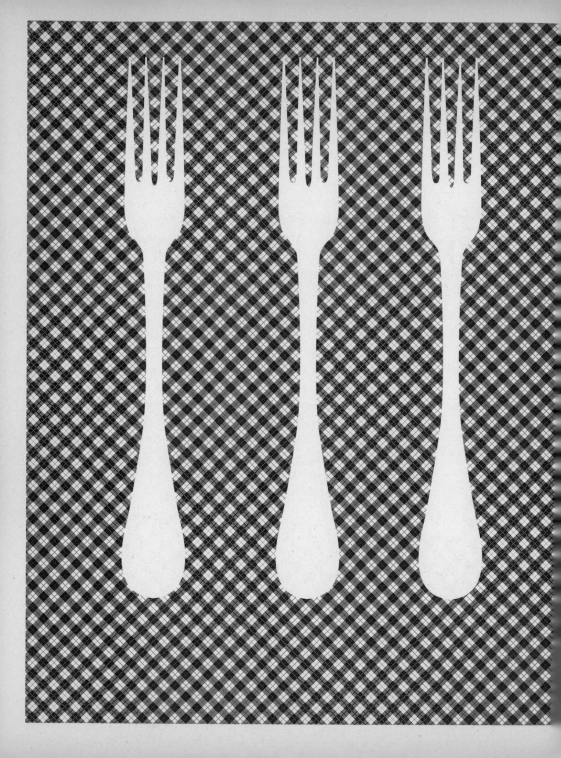

CHAPTER FOUR
HOW TO EAT PETITE
Part 1: What to Put on Your Fork

Now that you've hit Chapter Four, you're probably feeling a little peckish. It's way past teatime, right? Mercifully, there are easy, healthy ways to eat which keep one eye on moderation and the other on the scales. What you need is consciousness. Awareness.

A bit of Zen. Think before you drink, look before you eat. You don't need to make a song and dance about it – just be conscious of your intake. It's the smart, sustainable method of controlling calories, and not a diet in sight.

30 DRINK MORE SOUP

This is a stunningly simple way to eat less and still get a warm, full feeling in your bones. Soup, according to research from Penn State University, is a great appetite suppressant because it consists of a hunger-busting combination of liquids and solids; simply have it before a meal (in the traditional way) and you can lower your overall calorie intake by up to 20 per cent compared to a meal without soup.

But there's more. Having a wholesome, humble soup for lunch rather than buying your usual sandwich could have an even more dramatic effect on your waistline. According to the National Consumer Council, many of the flamboyant sandwiches on sale in high-street chains – the ones that look as if they could do a back-flip, make a coin appear from your cleavage and deliver a witty punchline – contain fiercely high levels of fat and salt. Pret à Manger's indisputably delicious dry-cured ham, cheese and mustard sandwich, for example, clocks in at 584 calories. A Big Mac, by contrast, contains 495 calories. Go figure.

You do need to be eating the right kind of soup, though. Some years ago, I decided to take the soup idea to the bridge by ditching lunch completely and replacing it with a tasty Slim-a-Soup instead. My favourite Chicken and Mushroom flavour, which I consumed for an entire fortnight, contained 1.7 per cent mushroom and 1.1 per cent chicken – less than its content of mono-potassium phosphate (an acidity regulator), and less still than E471 (an emulsifier). This, I soon found, was not a satisfying axis to a day. By three p.m. I would be ready to gnaw the door (luckily, I generally had a bag of Haribo Starmix to hand). Hopeless. The Cabbage Soup Diet is similarly vile, about as appetizing as a warm-fish milkshake, and – given its vicious odour and gas-promoting properties – a startlingly effective way to lose friends and alienate people.

What you really need is an honest, *nourishing* soup, preferably with some protein in it (beans and lentils will do the trick). In a perfect world, you'd probably make your own, having first produced a fine stock from heritage vegetables grown in your walled garden.

I am honestly thrilled for you if you inhabit such a world, but if not, the ready-made chilled soups you find in delis and supermarkets come a decent second. Look on the label to see how heavy-going it really is. As a rule, cheesy soups, 'cream-of' soups and meat-fest soups are full of gratuitous calories and aren't a patch on veggie broths. Go for delicate infusions – perhaps a Vietnamese Pho, with a kick of chilli, a fling of noodles and masses of coriander. Try borscht, consommé, la garbure and miso (stacked with essential amino acids, vitamins and minerals) over chowder, bisque and potage. If you have to use a knife and fork, you've lost the advantage.

If you're going to DIY, soups demand a pleasing seasonal approach, and are a deft destination for leftovers. Improvise (though please don't do what my husband once did and produce Roast Lunch Soup, using every last scrap from Sunday whizzed up in a blender). Do, however, play. Chuck an egg and some minuscule quadretti pasta into well-seasoned, densely flavoured chicken stock to make 'pasta in brodo', a low-key, fun-filled favourite of my childhood. Root about in the bottom of the fridge for forgotten vegetables – the leftover butternut squash, the past-it parsnips, a few tired carrots. Soft boil in stock, throw in any handy herbs and a scatter of chilli flakes, then blend and devour. Heaven in a bowl (and it will never taste the same twice, so much more than can be said of a Big Mac or an M&S prawn sandwich, which taste identical worldwide, regardless of your coordinates).

Avoid serving with a hunk o' bread or croutons or crackers (or Gruyère, aioli, rouille, dumplings . . .). But you knew that already. In summer, make it cool cucumber soup, green pea and mint, or zingy gazpacho. When cooking for friends, kick off a meal with a light brothy starter – it will fill you right up and ensure that you don't pig out when the main course rolls around.

As you sup, dwell upon the further evidence that you are doing yourself a whole lot of good: a two-year French study of five thousand individuals found that those who had soup five or six times a week were more likely to have BMIs below 23 (that's lean), compared with infrequent- or non-soup-drinkers, whose BMIs tended to be way up in the 27 range . . .

SLUUURP!
HOW TO DRINK SOUP IN POLITE COMPANY

✳ Spoon in a gentle motion away from the table edge.

✳ Fill the spoon three-quarters full.

✳ Scrape excess from the base of the spoon using the bowl.

✳ Turn to your right and enter into engaging conversation with the vicar.

✳ Don't blow. Wait.

✳ Do not put the entire spoon in your mouth; drink instead from the side of the spoon

✳ Ssshh! Not so loud.

✳ You may, if you wish, tilt the bowl away from you to scoop up the dregs, but don't do this more than twice or you will seem ungraciously ravenous, like Oliver or Tiny Tim.

✳ Rest the spoon in the bowl between mouthfuls. Do not rest it on the tablecloth, where it will make a dreadful stain, for which the hostess may bill you.

✳ When done, do not mop up with bread. What's done is done.

✳ *Vogue's Etiquette Guide* has the following to say about the final act: 'When one has finished one's soup, the spoon is left in the soup plate, handle to the right, over the edge of the plate, parallel to the edge of the table; but it should never be left in a soup cup or any other cup. The spoon should lie on the saucer of the cup. Never, even for a moment, should a spoon be left sticking out of the cup.'

✳ Ignore this. Soup in a cup is a glorious thing, second only to hot chocolate in a mug, and should be enjoyed with abandon. Soup in a basket is less successful. Soup in a flask is, by the way, the perfect portable meal.

31 GET FRESH AND FEEL THE FORCE

If your idea of a balanced diet is a cookie in each hand, it's clearly time to reset your dial. Plenty of people – whether seven-stone whips or seventeen-stone whoppers – are malnourished because they fail to eat sufficiently nutritious food. If you want to feel great and look incredible, you have to eat well, which means a varied diet with plenty of fresh stuff. Not exactly a shock revelation, I know, but stop griping. Put down those cookies and climb on board. Here are six sure-fire ways to increase your vitamin content:

✱ **Eating seasonal – and local – food helps**. Studies have confirmed what your heart already knows: that modern crop-breeding, accelerated growth, prolonged storage and long-distance transport lower the nutritional value of food. So stand on your doorstep. Try to eat things from within a twenty-five-mile radius; if you're in a vast metropolis, make it forty miles and pamper yourself with the knowledge that you're doing the planet a favour too. A little investigation should yield a prodigious harvest – whether it's local cheese, fresh fish or orchard fruits – wherever you're based.

Eating in this honest, grounded way may leave you feeling like a heroine in a Hardy novel, but let's be frank: fitting such Elysian bliss into a busy life is undoubtedly a challenge. I recently spent an entire weekend picking blackberries from nearby fields and turning them into bramble jelly; at ten o'clock on Sunday night, I realized we hadn't had any *lunch* and the kids' school uniforms were still trapped in the dirty-clothes basket nursing last week's grass stains. Clearly, we can't all know the family tree of the apples in our bowl. But we can make a stab at eating seasonally. Strawberries in December, as everyone knows, should be shot on sight. If your asparagus comes from Peru, and you don't, it's time to alter your feeding habits.

✱ **Uncook! Go raw!** You'll lose weight, for sure, since bite for bite vegetables and fruit generally have fewer calories than processed foods. They boast a high water content, are rich in fibre and haven't lost any of the vitamins and vitality that can be killed in cooking. What's more, research shows you may well live longer too. This is, of course, fabulous news for hopeless cooks across the land. The idea is that nothing should be heated beyond 118°F, the point at which vital enzymes and nutrients can be destroyed. As David Wolfe, America's leading raw-food guru, puts it: 'The psychedelic feeling of pure joy that one derives from eating high-quality raw foods cannot be compared to anything one has experienced before . . . Inner cleanliness is an exquisite feeling! On top of this, raw plant food gives you superhuman powers!' Yes, all that from alfalfa sprouts!

My dear friend Pen swears by the mystic power of her shredded-beetroot salad. It may sound a bit low-key, but it is sublime when you shuttle it into your mouth:

For four people, coarsely grate three medium-sized fresh beetroot (just scrub under water, there's no need to peel – wear rubber gloves to avoid staining your hands; and the grating must be coarse otherwise the beetroot will become slushy).

Grate three carrots using the same large holes on your grater. Add a quarter of celeriac if you feel like it, or some grated apple. Mix the following to make a dressing:

> 2 tbsps horseradish sauce
> 2 tbsps olive oil
> 1 tbsp freshly squeezed lemon or orange juice
> 1 tsp English mustard
> A garlic clove or two, diced, chopped, squashed,
>   or not at all if you are about to go on a date
> Salt and pepper to taste

Dress the grated veggies and top with sesame or pumpkin seeds.

If you want some protein with that, give *crudo* a go – an Italian version of sushi. The tissue-thin raw fish – bass, bream, mackerel – is served with olive oil, lemon juice and fresh herbs rather than wasabi, soy sauce and a shaving of pickled ginger.

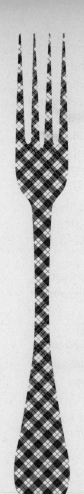

✶ **Have it handy**. If you're a bit Bree, keep a selection of crunchy crudités ready-cut in iced water in the fridge. If you're a bit me, have an apple in your drawers. Keep fruit available, looking charming in a bowl, not exhausted beyond resuscitation in the bottom of the fridge. Pears, as Eddie Izzard noted, are particularly rubbish in this respect: 'They're gorgeous little beasts, but they're ripe for *half an hour*, and you're never there. They're like a rock, or they're mush . . . you put them in the bowl at home, and they sit there, going, "No! No! Don't ripen yet, don't ripen yet. Wait till he goes out the room! Ripen! *Now, now, now!*"' It may be worth persevering with pears, though, watching them like a hawk for that brief moment of perfection: researchers at the State University of Rio de Janeiro have found that overweight women who ate three small pears a day lost more weight on a low-calorie diet than women who didn't add fruit to their diet . . .

✶ **Buy good, green, fresh herbs**, not dried ones – and house olive oil in an air-tight, darkened container to keep it vital and vibrant.

✶ **Think whole**. In the past, I have always found hempy wholefood stores a mild turn-off. I only needed to stand in the aisle to be plagued with guilt. 'I'm not Amnesty enough,' my soul would yell. 'I didn't recycle the honey jar.' My leather shoes would step over the threshold and shout their provenance and price. 'We're dead cows!' they'd shriek. 'Expensive dead cows!' Mercifully, I have since matured and got over the hump – partly because, thanks to the eco-revolution, the shops themselves have stepped out of the seventies. If you're not doing it already, it's well worth taking a regular weekly sweep around your local wholefood store to see what grabs your fancy – an aloe drink, perhaps, or a stick of unrefined liquorice. Whatever keeps you off factory food is fine by me.

✶ **Know that calcium counts**. Though dairy has long been the demon in the fridge for serial dieters, it turns out that calcium – one of milk's vital components – can help facilitate weight loss. In studies, people on a reduced-calorie diet who included some dairy foods lost significantly more weight than those who ate a low-dairy diet containing the same number of calories. Research at the University of Tennessee found that when fat cells are exposed to a calcium-rich environment, they break down fat more swiftly than in calcium-depleted conditions. If you want to boost your calcium intake without resorting to the fat-fest of Cheddar, go for the brilliance of broccoli. It is high in vitamin C too, which helps foster calcium absorption. If you're in a hurry, consider taking a calcium supplement.

32 TURN JAPANESE

You may already know that the Japanese have some of the lowest obesity rates in the developed world. While their traditionally low consumption of dairy is partly responsible for this enviable state of affairs (as is their use of chopsticks, which can slow down a feeding frenzy), their diet also owes much to food served in varying degrees of rawness, keeping it nutritionally sound and engagingly natural. The other key difference is that the Japanese tend to consume a good deal less meat than Westerners. According to the latest estimates from *The Economist*'s Intelligence Unit, Japanese people eat 45 kilos of meat per person per year. The US annual figure is 130 kilos, while in France it's 103 kilos, and in Great Britain a still-substantial 82 kilos. The average Briton manages just one-third of a portion of fish a week. Shame on us. Fish is high in protein and low in saturated fat (unless you drown it in batter and fry it in a bottomless well of oil). What's more, salmon, mackerel, eel – the oily fish – are admirably high in Omega 3 essential fatty acids, which will help you with sudoku when you are elderly, making them ideal dinner guests.

Eating fish in the raw retains its nutrients. If turning Japanese, go for sashimi over sushi (no rice!) and make sure it's as fresh as a lively breeze off the Solent (it's amazing what the hot kiss of wasabi can do for a sliver of naked salmon). If raw leaves you cold and you need a 'cooked' flavour, try *ceviche*. The acid in the citrus juice will 'cook' the fish without heat, turning it from translucent to opalescent before your very eyes. This is a traditional Latin American method, and requires (of course) the freshest fish you can muster. It works with bass, cod, mackerel – but is particularly good with snapper, and even better eaten on deck with a very cold beer. Here's how:

> 1 red snapper fillet (or preferred fish) per person, boned, skinned and cubed into half-inch pieces
> Juice of a lime, juice of a lemon
> Diced red onion – you decide how much or if at all
> 1 red chilli, deseeded and finely chopped
> A little salt, a grind of pepper, a hint of Tabasco to taste
> A suggestion of fresh grated root ginger would be good
> A fistful of coriander, loosely chopped

Place all the ingredients in a non-reactive bowl and eat within minutes, or put in the fridge for a few hours, stirring very occasionally, or whenever you happen to be visiting for a beer.

There are caveats to eating more fish, though. Be aware of conflicting advice about the 'safe' amount of fish to consume. While the FDA (Food and Drug Administration in the States) and the FSA (Food Standards Agency in the UK) recommend a limit of two portions of fish a week to avoid over-exposure to potential pollutants, other health experts advocate three portions a week to maximize genuine health benefits. You should rely on your common sense to arrive at an amount that works best for you.

If you are more concerned about the sustainability issue, choose stocks which have been certified by the Marine Stewardship Council (Pacific cod, hand-raked clams, Dover sole, Thames herring, Cornish sea bass and so on. For the full low-down, get hold of the Marine Conservation Society's Good Fish Guide at fishonline.org).

If you want to combine all your concerns in one goodly little fish, look to Cornish sardines or pilchards: loaded with protein, high in Omega 3, cheap as chips, and impressively light in contaminants since they live low on the food chain. Go for sardines caught in traditional drift or ring nets and you've got yourself a very fine fish, especially if you brush them with herby, garlicky olive oil and sling them on searing hot charcoal.

33 BUY MORE FOOD THAT HAS NO LABEL

Make a point of choosing fresh produce with a coating of earth, not cellophane. I know it's hardly a scoop to tell you that you'd do better to eat food as nature intended – but let's just say that I'm covering all bases here. If your potatoes are croquettes and your chicken is nuggets, not only are you doing your mouth a disservice, you're doing your waistline no good at all.

So go naked (it's apparently how Nicole Kidman maintains her enviable figure: 'She has healthy eating habits,' says a friend. 'She's very picky about what goes in her mouth – she doesn't eat anything from a box or a can'). This should apply to most of what ends up in your shopping trolley, and not only the fresh stuff. Products which don't require much in the way of packaging tend to feature fewer stabilizers, additives or E-numbers. You could even make it yourself . . .

HOW VERY CULTURED:
WHY DIY YOGHURT IS SUBLIME

I don't want to freak you out, but what's to stop you making your own yoghurt? It's not beyond you, and yoghurt is an all-round, calcium-rich, protein-fuelled wonder-food – even though I stopped eating the stuff for a decade from the age of eight because my friend Eddie Wall told me that yoghurt was alive and if you listened closely you could hear it scream. I listened closely and spent my formative years with yoghurt in my hair as a result. Never once heard it scream though.

Before Eddie Wall ruined it, yoghurt played a big part in my little life. One of my keenest childhood memories is the leaf-green Thermos my mother kept for the express purpose of making yoghurt. It would sit on a sill, alive with promise, until time was up and she'd spoon out great quivering white dollops of fresh, tangy deliciousness, easily as good as Angel Delight (as long as you were allowed to add a slick of golden syrup). While you can produce the stuff in a yoghurt-maker, the art of doing it in an airing cupboard, in an old Thermos, is one which is well worth revisiting on a lazy, rainy day. Here's what to do:

✳ Sterilize your milk (any milk – you choose) by heating to *near* boiling; stir to avoid scorching.

✳ Cool – you can put the saucepan in a sink half-filled with cold water.

✳ Stir in a couple of tablespoons of your groovy live culture. This can be any shop-bought yoghurt which boasts 'active cultures', or – for greater reliability – go for specialist freeze-dried bacteria, available online, or at the wholefood store where you are now known by name.

✳ Pour into leaf-green Thermos or similar.

✳ Incubate, perhaps in the airing cupboard, or on a sunny window ledge.

✳ It will thicken in a day. Stick it in the fridge.

✳ Reserve enough to beget your next batch. (Don't you love this generational thing? It's almost biblical!)

✳ Adorn the rest with fresh raspberries, chopped hazelnuts and a drizzle – yes, go on then – of golden syrup.

34 RETRAIN YOUR PALATE, WAKE UP YOUR MOUTH

Fed up with your fridge? Jaded by the tedium of your kitchen cupboards? Does a shiftless apathy envelop you at the prospect of supper? Well, same here. Deciding what to cook, as any householder knows, is an abominable drag. Personally, I'm happy to shop, chop, cook and clean up afterwards, I may even throw in a song and dance routine – so long as someone tells me what to serve. There is no earthly point wandering hopelessly around the supermarket sniffing for inspiration. You will emerge momentarily triumphant, only to find you have come home with a large pie and three different types of pasta. Better by far to know in advance at least some of the meals you're likely to consume over the next week or so.

Rather than rely on old standbys and faithful favourites, you'd do well to mix it up a bit. The Japanese, for instance, aim for five colours at each meal: red, blue-green, yellow, white and black. Give it a go, and your vegetable intake will soar. Ancient Ayurveda, meanwhile, recommends that the key to a satisfying meal lies in the inclusion of all six basic tastes (sweet, sour, salty, bitter, pungent and astringent). Pish? Perhaps. But a rounded, varied plate of food is bound to fill you and thrill you far more than a pizza, where every bite tastes broadly the same unless you happen upon a jalapeno. As a rule, if one food group covers your entire plate, you're barking up the wrong tree.

Develop a loose repertoire of evening meals that are hasty, tasty, but above all low in fats and fast-release carbs. Write them down. Keep the list in your purse, not stuck to the fridge. (Who brings a fridge to the shops?) Don't think of it as a menu plan, don't stick to it like glue, don't have it laminated and peer at it each morning saying, 'Ah, Tuesday! Must be tofu kebabs.' But do think ahead, just a bit. Have a broad idea when you are trolling around Sainsbury's of the kind of low-effort cooking that won't sink your ship. My favourites include:

✳ **OK Fish**. I've always called it this because it hails from the kitchen of our friends the O'Kellys, who live in the lee of the South Downs surrounded by children and chickens. The idea is to chuck it all in the oven (the ingredients, not the children and the chickens, God forbid) Jamie Oliver style, and see what deliciousness emerges. It's different every time, and you have to be fond of olives right from the off, but OK Fish is always wholesome and hearty, cunningly dispensing with the usual carbo-loading you get from your average British supper. So don't go mopping up the juices with a great wodge of bread, there's a dear.

> A packet of fine green beans; blanch first in boiling water
> A sheaf of asparagus, blanched. Broccoli works too
> Some cherry tomatoes. Chuck in the vine as well for flavour
> Greek olives – the black wizened ones, not Kalamata
> A good slosh of extra-virgin olive oil
> A lemon, squeezed. The peel goes in the pan too
> Salmon – a fillet per person – seasoned with rock salt and
>   coarse pepper and placed on top of the veggies
> Chilli flakes optional. Herbs like coriander, thyme or dill
>   are equally optional

Oven-cook in a roasting tin at 200°C for 20 minutes, or until the fish is cooked to your liking. Serve. Eat. Smile.

✳ **Tuna Fagioli.** This was one of the nonchalant little Italian suppers I grew up on, when everyone else was having gammon topped with pineapple followed by Arctic Roll. These days, it seems to me to be the perfect supper – comfortingly low in all the things you ought to avoid, but high in boundless flavour. It is simplicity itself to prepare, a real store-cupboard standby, and – like chilli con carne – it tastes even better on Day Two. Use an excellent olive oil (the price is your guide. Sorry, but it is. Same goes for shoes – what do you want me to say?). The classic fagioli uses cannellini beans, but you can mix and match. Try kidney beans, aduki, black-eye, whatever. I add a generous squeeze of lemon juice to mine, together with a fistful of torn flat-leaf parsley – not strictly the old-time Florentine recipe, but all the more delicious for it.

> 1 drained tin tuna (in brine – no need to add second-rate oil to this dish)
> 2 tins beans, drained
> 1 red onion, thinly sliced or chopped
> Juice of half a lemon
> 1 crushed garlic clove
> 2 glugs good olive oil
> 2 tbsps white wine vinegar
> Flat-leaf parsley, torn
> Rock salt and freshly ground pepper

Put everything in a bowl. Mix it up. Eat it, or stick it in the fridge for later. Serve with those fat red tomatoes – ones which really taste tomatoey, as if they are the distilled essence of a hot Tuscan day – quartered, salted, olive-oiled and demolished.

What else? There are other great recipes which are bang on the money in terms of calories, but rammed with ramped-up flavour. You'll have your own hit-list, but here are a few more of mine:

✻ **Oriental chicken salad**. Oven-cook four chicken breasts. Rest. Tear to shreds. Dress with a generous handful of coriander and mint leaves, chopped spring onion, olive oil, 1 tbsp Thai fish sauce, 1 tsp sesame oil, 2 limes, juiced. Season and serve on a crunchy bed of iceberg lettuce and cucumber crescents, dousing the lot in the remaining dressing.

✻ **Tuna Niçoise**. I boil baby new potatoes, eggs and fine green beans in the same saucepan (once boiling, the beans come out on a slotted spoon after five minutes, the eggs after ten and the potatoes after fifteen). Cool it all, with the hard-boiled eggs plunged into ice-cold water to prevent the yolks greying. Build a substantial nest of dressed leaves in a splendid bowl; add cherry tomatoes, seeds, olives, anchovies to taste, then the chilled beans, potatoes and quartered eggs. Sear seasoned tuna steaks (one each), quickly enough to retain a pale-pink interior – not more than a few minutes in a hot griddle pan. Squeeze with lemon as they cook, rest, then place precariously, deliciously, on the waiting salad. Add lemon wedges, coarse pepper and a glitter of sea salt. Spectacular. Up your bean-to-potato ratio to max out the good stuff, or, better still, skip the potatoes altogether – there's more than enough going on here without the need for them. A tin of tuna works perfectly well if you haven't got the fresh (and far more expensive) stuff.

✸ **Beef carpaccio** – raw and sliced ultra-thin – with rocket leaves. Good beef. Good rocket. Lemon. Olive oil. The usual.

✸ **Buffalo mozzarella**, prosciutto, tomatoes (more of those tasty ones) and basil, drizzled with olive oil and A-grade balsamic.

✸ **Smoked trout**, shredded into low-fat crème fraiche. Add crunchy sliced celeriac and horseradish to taste and serve with interesting leaves. A cos, perhaps.

✸ **Omelette** with chilli and onions, not cheese and ham.

✸ **Grilled cod** with steamed green vegetables. Sugar snaps, tender-stem broccoli, asparagus. All good.

✸ **Smoked haddock** with poached egg and a wilted heap of young spinach leaves (drain everything well on kitchen roll; your food should flirt, not float).

✸ **A whole baked fish** – sea bass, say – with herbs in its belly and salsa verde on the side.

✸ **Endive leaves** with fresh pear and walnuts, spiked with a crumble of Roquefort.

✸ **Mezze**. Award yourself small taste tests of – ooh, I don't know – tart, pipped olives, coarse hummus, fingers of wholemeal pitta. Add a tang of feta cheese, some semi-dried tomatoes, a dollop of aubergine dip, sticks of celery, red pepper and carrot, artichoke hearts, tangy pickled shallots. Or go Greek with the classic cucumber-tomato-red-onion-feta combo, drizzled in extra-virgin and a squeeze of lemon.

35 CHOOSE FAT-BURNERS, NOT FATS

Some foods demand that you eat more. They chivvy and tease, they breed cravings and hankerings, they gaze at you from the open packet and invite you to have *just one more* ('You can't Sara Lee-ve them alone', 'Once you pop you can't stop', 'Made to make your mouth water', 'Betcha can't eat just one'...). Thus ensnared, your blood sugar bounces about like a beach ball, and – bang – you're down to the last Pringle before you've had time to un-notch your belt.

Other foods, by divine contrast, satisfy. They contain clever components which can stimulate a metabolism or rev up your day. These nutrient-rich foods are considered by many to be almost magical in their capacity to crush hunger and speed up your body's fat-burning power. Here, listed in no particular order, are nine flab-busting, fat-burning foods (and why they work). Don't panic. You don't need to eat them all at every meal. You are not Gwyneth Paltrow, and this is not a fad diet regime. But try to introduce them to your plate from time to time. Choose these at the expense of their less effective brethren. And keep that belt notched up.

✳ **Grapefruit**. No, no, no, *not* the Grapefruit Diet, which requires you to go about your daily business in the constant companionship of a couple of grapefruit, your only respite being the occasional pink one or perhaps a nice glass of grapefruit juice. To depend so heavily on a single foodstuff is both dull and disastrous. BUT there is some evidence to suggest that grapefruit is a kick-ass fat-fighter. Researchers at the Scripps Clinic in La Jolla, California, have investigated its effect on weight loss and found that eating half a grapefruit before a meal can indeed help. Though not quite nailed yet, the theory suggests there is a physiological link between grapefruit and a reduction in insulin levels, which serves to impede fat storage. What's more, grapefruit contains cancer-fighting compounds such as liminoids and lycopene, and clocks in at only 39 calories per hemisphere.

✳ **Apples**. The humble apple really is worth keeping about your person. Not only is it a portable, pre-packed powerhouse, loaded with vitamin C, fibre, sustaining sugars and crunch, it is – if you shop wisely – likely to be a more local product than a banana, with all the health and environmental benefits that brings. Apples are also a superb source of pectin, a soluble fibre which can't be absorbed by the body, but can be very handy on its way through. Pectin makes the apple a fiercely functional food: it is thought to limit the amount of fat your cells can absorb, it helps to balance blood-sugar levels and can even cause the stomach to empty more slowly, leaving you fuller longer. In addition to all this good stuff, pectin was recently found to have anti-carcinogenic effects in the colon. What's more, there is also something aesthetically pleasing about an apple: its rounded heft in your hand, the roses on its cheeks, its ability to simultaneously explain the laws of gravity and dance with cloves in a pie. I'll give you six kiwis for a single orange pippin any day.

✳ **Olive oil**. Scientists have recently discovered that oleic acid – a fatty acid found in abundance in olive oil, though also present in nuts and avocados – can trigger a reaction in the body that staves off hunger pangs. It is converted by the digestive system into a hormone called oleoylethanolamide: tricky to spell, yes, but a powerful no-diet dieting tool which will keep you satisfied between meals in a way that a bag of Skittles never could.

✳ **Flax seeds**. A tiny, insubstantial sort of seed, true, but flax is a potent cocktail of edible goodies. Its scientific name, *Linum usitatissimum*, means 'most useful' – and a brief saunter through its benefits proves why: flax seeds have been shown to help control high blood pressure, promote bone health, lower cholesterol and – important to us – boost the metabolism, which can help stimulate weight loss. These tiddly seeds are rich in alpha linolenic acid (that's an Omega-3 fat) and they are a condensed source of anti-viral, antioxidant lignans, together with all manner of vitamins and minerals, and, as a final parting shot, system-sweeping fibre. They taste vaguely nutty and are a superior addition to your morning cereal or porridge. Use the cold-pressed oil for salad dressings (don't cook with it or you'll annihilate the goodness).

✶ **Lecithin**. It might sound like a man-made nutraceutical (Eat Less! Be thin! With Lecithin™!), but it is in fact a vital component of your body. Approximately a third of the 'dry weight' of your brain – I know, *eeeuch*, but bear with me here – is formed of the stuff. Lecithin is a fat-like substance produced in the liver, essential for making each cell's protective membrane, thus responsible for the control of nutrients in and out, like a bouncer at Boujis. It is high in B vitamins, particularly choline, which is blessed with a detergent-like ability to break up fats. Beyond the science, all you really need to know is that lecithin is a good guy. You can find it in soya beans, eggs (the word itself is derived from the Greek word *likithos*, meaning egg yolk), grains and brewer's yeast. It is your fat shield. Wear it well.

✶ **Garlic**. In laboratory tests on rats, scientists at Israel's Weizmann Institute of Science found that garlic apparently prevents weight gain and, though the process is still only partially understood, may even lead to weight loss. As far as I'm aware, they didn't test it as a vampire-repellent – but, really, I wouldn't be surprised if it could do that too. Garlic is, says biochemist David Mirelman, a 'wonder drug', brilliant at a whole range of jobs, from lowering blood pressure to treating diabetes – thanks to its active ingredient allicin. It is this sulphurous compound which gives garlic its pungency, and, it is thought, protects cells and reduces fatty deposits. Even if you don't buy the bumf, it's worth noting the hallowed place reserved for garlic in history. It helped build the pyramids; it powered Greek athletes; it protected Roman centurions; Hippocrates himself recommended garlic for infections, wounds, leprosy and digestive disorders. I recommend it for spaghetti puttanesca. Or bake it whole in its skin alongside a roast.

✱ **Blueberries**. In the pantheon of super-foods (small yawn), few are as comely and toothsome as the blueberry. These mega berries are powerfully antioxidant, and rammed with sparkling vitamin C – which, as you'll recall from Point Eleven, is a vital tool for weight management.

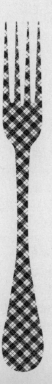

✱ **Almonds**. It's always worth remembering that the food industry is well versed in promoting its products as wonder, super, über and otherwise heroic. But if you are to believe the hype, almonds are pretty much the food of the gods. Forget milk and honey. Eat almonds. For years, scientists have been vaguely aware that people who regularly eat almonds tend to weigh less than people who don't. No one was entirely sure why or how – until a series of studies started to unveil their secrets. One, from Purdue University in Indiana, found that adding two servings of almonds to an existing diet had no effect on body weight or percentage of body fat per se, but *did* satisfy hunger rather brilliantly. The researchers also found that the fibre in almonds seemed to block some of the fat they contain from being digested and absorbed. To top it all, preliminary research from the University of Toronto suggests that eating almonds can reduce the impact that carb-rich food has on blood-sugar levels. Too good to be true? Who knows? My feeling, in a nutshell, is give them a go. They're protein-packed, nutritious, high in fibre; they don't smell, they don't leak and they fit neatly (I have discovered) into the interior pocket of an Hermès Kelly bag.

✱ **Sunflower seeds**. Stacked with good fats. And iron, zinc, potassium, fibre, vitamins E and B1, magnesium, selenium . . . I could go on, but the big sell is that they take *ages* to eat, if you go for the unshelled variety. A whole evening can be gone and you've only consumed seven seeds, working like a meadow pipit for every last scrap. Genius.

36 THROW OUT THE FRYING PAN AND BUY A FIVE-LEVEL STEAMER

Simply going from fried to grilled and using a steamer will save so many calories that you'll fall off your chair. If you fancy chips, don't open a frosty packet and pour them into a deep-fat fryer; chop up a potato and stick the wedges in a roasting tin with a snatch of rosemary and a dash of olive oil. Rather then building an entire meal in a frying pan, build *up*, not out, in a multi-storey steamer. Start on the ground floor with a delicate fillet of white fish, then mangetouts in the next storey up, and a handful of young spinach in the penthouse. Again, small things, big calorie savings. Do some DIY and get building.

37 SURVIVE THE SNACK ATTACKS

I'm not a harridan. I know that you may need to keep your ghrelin in check with the occasional snack. Fine. But if you really must graze, do it mindfully and find a tasty low-cal treat which works for you. Rather than endless snacking on foods developed in test tubes and tested on rats, go natural. According to Hollywood lore, a good many A-listers rely on asparagus and parsley as snacks, because they believe these morsels repress hunger and reduce bloating (actually, they don't work, though they are mildly diuretic and may make you feel momentarily lighter). Nor is there any real need to go mad and have a handful of raisins like Elizabeth Hurley or a few sugar-snap peas like Victoria Beckham. Try the following instead:

✳ **Be prepared**. Don't leave the house hungry, or you will walk blindly towards the nearest bun shop. Keep an apple in your handbag (see Point Thirty-five to know why). My great friend Valerie always carries a boiled egg in her Mulberry Bayswater, but then she is a trifle odd.

✱ **Wow your mouth** with the occasional taste treat. It's your mouth, you decide. At the moment (and you may well find them disagreeable), I'm going with Fisherman's Friend Cherry Menthols – a bomblet of curiously punchy flavour contained in a humble three-calorie lozenge which you find on the counter at chemists, alongside the vitamin C tablets and the strawberry-flavoured condoms. I'm also partial to the occasional Proctor's Pinelyptus Pastille, a gloriously yesteryear idea, 'as used by Lords, Ladies, Principal Public Speakers, Singers and Members of Parliament, for Clarity of Voice'. You might prefer an orange Tic Tac. Or that chewing gum which is so full of menthol flavour that it makes your eyes water and your hair stand on end. Whatever it is, the idea is to flirt with your mouth from time to time – giving it powerful hits of taste – so that it doesn't lead you into temptation. Better a Tic Tac than three rounds of Marmite toast.

✱ **Pack in the packets**. You don't need a PhD in nutrition to work out that you should try to snack on things that *grow* – olives, blueberries, cornichons, baby beetroot, seeds of any and all descriptions, plum tomatoes, cucumber sticks, carrot batons. Keep them close. Dip them in hummus or tzatziki if you have to. In a pretty little bowl, right here in front of my keyboard, I have cherry tomatoes on the vine (their fragrance reminds me of the intense tang of my grandmother's greenhouse in high summer, the air thick with heat and the thrum of insects, the tomato plants giving off their wild green perfume). I've also got a handful of fat pink radishes – those long ones that look like they're blushing – and some bright-white cauliflower florets cold from the fridge. I know it's not millionaire's shortbread, but it does fill that snacky gap you get when you're working, when your jaw is bored and your stomach is not exactly demanding lunch, but suggesting that it could do with a moment of attention.

✱ **Eat heat**. Avoid bland foods and snack instead on fiery pickles, hot chillis and strong flavours that your brain will remember. (I'm into piquillo peppers at the moment; grown in northern Spain, these babies are hand-picked, roasted over an open fire, peeled and packed in their own juices in a jar.) You might prefer Manzanilla olives stuffed with a salty kick of anchovy, sweet pickled Guindilla chillies, or skinny slivers of paprika chorizo. As you nibble on these passionate snacks, amuse yourself with the news that researchers at Laval University in Canada have recently found that eating hot peppers can speed up your metabolism, cool your cravings and lower your calorie intake. Apparently, capsaicin – a compound found in jalapeno and cayenne peppers – 'temporarily stimulates your body to release more stress hormones, which speeds up your metabolism and causes you to burn more calories'. Ginger, mixed spice and black pepper are thought to have similar thermogenic effects, according to research at Maastricht University. So fire 'em up.

✶ **As a last resort** . . . If you must, have a Jaffa Cake. Though they contain sugar and, of course, calories, they are relatively low in fat (1g per cake). This does turn into 8g per 100g, so don't get to the last crumb of one and embark on another. You will, however, have just enjoyed an illusion of fat, housed in a whole heap of taste. Otherwise, go for . . .

✶ **Home-popped popcorn**. Madonna's snack of choice is equally cheeky but low in those devilish calories (so long as you don't lard it with butter, sugar or a combination of the two).

38 IF YOU'RE FEELING PECKISH, BRUSH YOUR TEETH

Works every time. If you brush your teeth after a meal, some folk – including Matthew McConaughey, apparently – believe that a new taste in the mouth sends a signal to the brain that you are full. It will also please your dentist.

39 ORDER ONE PUDDING, TWO FORKS

Twice the fun, half the calories. There are countless other clever ways to eat neat, of course:

* **Order two starters and no main.**

* **Take a vow of pudding abstinence**, with an amnesty every third Tuesday.

* **Choose fiddly foods** – lobster or crab, perhaps – which occupy hands and mouth, are fantastically sociable and suck up great fathoms of time. I've always found that there are few things as convivial as a platter of iced *fruits de mer* at Bofinger, in the rue de la Bastille, the oldest brasserie in Paris and the haunt of presidents and ministers, Chiracs and Chevaliers. A whole enjoyable evening can disappear and you still won't have started on the whelks.

* **Similarly, crispy Peking duck** in a Chinese restaurant is time-consuming and pleasing, engaging both conversation and the effort of many fingers.

* **Ditto artichokes**. So sociable – dip the leaves in vinaigrette, not melted butter.

* **And edamame soy beans from a sushi bar**, or indeed from a little ceramic bowl planted on your desk (just three grams of fat per 100 grams!). Though fiddly, satay, it should be noted, is less appealing on several counts: it's usually fried, it comes with a heavy-going peanut sauce and there is always the prospect that you will do as I once did in a very upmarket restaurant. Attempting to prise a chicken chunk from its stick, I applied rather too much force and a missile of meat flew across the room like a superhero and landed in the handbag of a fellow diner two tables away. She didn't notice. I didn't tell her. It feels so good to confess.

40 DON'T BE A TRASHIONISTA

I'm the first to adhere to the anonymous adage that 'there are four basic food groups: milk chocolate, dark chocolate, white chocolate and chocolate truffles'. We all know there are times in a life, and times of the month, when a little cocoa can go a long way towards making you feel loved and human and soft-centred again. No one is asking you to endure a Decaflon (according to the *Washington Post*, this is 'the gruelling event of getting through the day consuming only things that are good for you'). And don't straitjacket yourself with the cardiologist's diet ('If it tastes good, spit it out'); deprivation is, after all, no way to live a life – and that's what we're after here, remember: sustainable, permanent, attainable change. Fine. But when you *do* treat yourself, try a little bit of lovely, not a whole lot of junk. Make it a fantastic oozy Brie, not cheese on toast; a Chateau Chic, not a bottle of splosh; a couple of squares of Rococo geranium-infused chocolate; not, not, not a family bar of Mint Aero. And make sure that occasional treats stay occasional – otherwise, like Hansel and Gretel, you will be following a trail of tasty morsels all the way back to the old, fat you.

If you are going to have a periodic off-script splurge, you may as well go for things that have other benefits. For example:

✸ **Red wine**. Though relatively high in calories, the odd glass of vino rosso is also high in resveratrol, thought to boast a host of benefits – not least that it may offset the negative effects of gluttony. Studies at Maastricht University suggest that grapeseed extract can reduce calorie intake; meanwhile, researchers at the Harvard Medical School also found that resveratrol slows down the ageing process in non-mammalian animals. Doesn't necessarily mean it will work for you and me, but we'll give it a go shall we?

✸ **Butter**. Rather blissfully, butter contains conjugated linoleic acid, which is thought to help fight breast cancer. What a bonus. Even so, keep it as a treat, not a habit. Use olive oil or rapeseed oil for cooking, and have a little bit of butter sometimes. On Sunday, with hot toast and the papers.

✳ Proper chocolate. New research says that cocoa may well contain more antioxidants than green tea. And, as every ad exec knows, it is thought to have aphrodisiac and serotonin-boosting properties, which can certainly get a girl through a miserable Monday in one piece. As Gwyneth Paltrow confessed to *Grazia* magazine: 'Once in a while I'll have some good chocolate cake.' The operative words in this sentence are 'once' and 'good', not 'chocolate' and 'cake'. Remember that all chocolate contains fat and sugar, but some is fatter and sweeter than others. Always go for the top-drawer stuff. Perhaps something from Valrhona or Richart or Green and Black's. Either way, next time you bite into a Raspberry Ganache Twirl or a Dark Praline Crescent, don't think, 'Blimey, calories!' Think, 'Mmm, antioxidant flavonoids . . .'

And if you do occasionally fall off the wagon, treat it as a momentary hiccup, not a Greek tragedy. Move on. There are better things to do than mope. Like? Well, like reading the next chapter, for one.

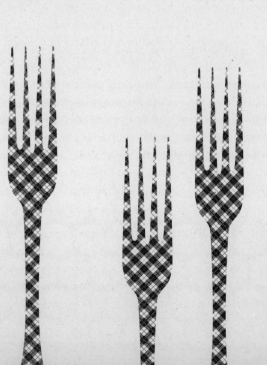

CHAPTER FIVE
HOW TO
DRESS THIN
. . . and Cheat the World

You've come a long way, baby. You've discovered ways to trim and pare, ways to think thin and eat smart. Now for the divinely easy part. You only want to diet because you think you look fat, right? So don't look fat! What you need is the fashion editor's inside track on diet dressing – all of those cunning, stunning little tricks that get your wardrobe to do the work, so you don't have to.

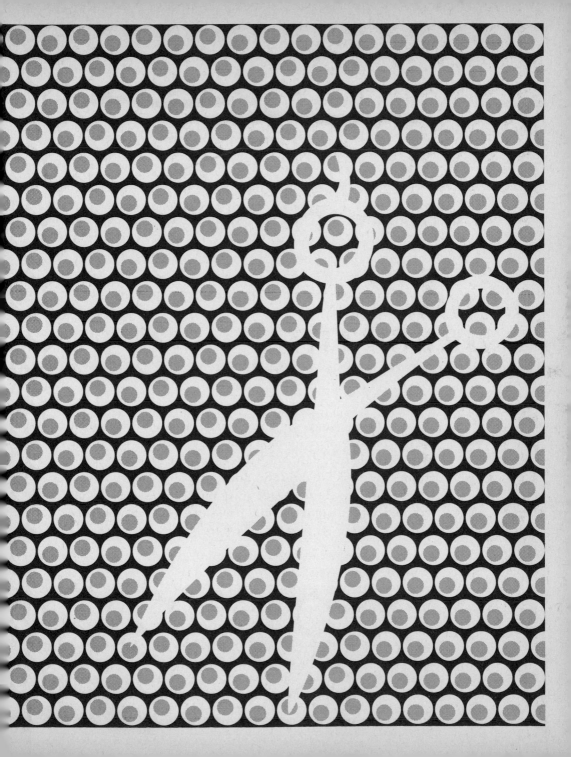

41   GET A DIET DRESS

As Mark Twain so neatly noted, 'Clothes make the man. Naked people have little or no influence in society.' Dead right, but what he omitted to add is that when it comes to the *woman*, clothes don't just make her. They can break her. It all hinges on the dozens of tiny decisions that flit through your barely conscious mind as you gaze into your closet of a morning. Should you risk the dungarees to take the kids to school? (Probably not.) Are culottes acceptable for a meeting with your estate agent? (Possibly, if you'd like him to show you properties with corner baths.) Can you take your cleavage to church? (Yes, but make it wear a scarf.)

Getting it wrong is a constant threat – a botheration that barely afflicts men, who know that a suit, by and large, will get them through any scenario without unduly troubling the eye. But we women need clothes we can trust, clothes we can rely on in a storm or a heatwave, clothes that will take us gently by the hand and lead us through thick and thin and all manner of tribulations in between. And most of all, most of us, most of the time, need a Diet Dress.

This fabled garment is the absolute axis of a slimline life, and though its specifics are wholly personal, there are a handful of rules which apply to us all. A Diet Dress's success is almost all in the cut, which is why it's worth spending both time and money on its purchase. There are designers who, having studied the arc and arch of the female form, are a dab hand at cutting a Diet Dress. By way of example, Alber Elbaz, designer at Lanvin, cuts a superlative sleeveless dress, which somehow manages to conceal the ugly under-arm swag we all despise. Perhaps you love your arms, but hate your sloping shoulders? In which case, look for a little padding in the area to give you a lift. You might want to rediscover your waist or entertain the idea of a bracelet sleeve, the better to show off an elegant wrist. It doesn't really matter what it is: the point is, you and you alone must find your asset and invest in it.

Though it works admirably hard, clocking up hour after hour on duty, the Diet Dress should be the unobtrusive element in your wardrobe – not the wicked, foxy, thrusty number that introduces itself to strangers at parties. Not the one that everybody will notice and remember next time it gets an outing. Not the one that makes you think about it every third minute, like a newborn infant, demanding your attention because it has risen up your thigh or dipped down to reveal your bra strap. No. A Diet Dress is the strong and silent type. Reliable. Quietly confident.

Its shape will depend, largely, on yours. My own Diet Dress is in a delicious midnight-blue silk jersey, the colour of deep water. It is high at the neck – a surprise to me, that – with an asymmetric hem, bell sleeves and a dropped waist. If this sounds hideous, well, hands off, it's mine. The point is that this particular dress makes *me* feel fabulous. And, perhaps more to the point, it makes me feel thin. It is lengthy and languid, elongating rather than widening my body. It clings in all the right places and tactfully skims over the wrong ones, and it is my Diet Dress chiefly because of the body that inhabits it. Your Diet Dress will probably be another species entirely. It may feature something sturdy in the bodice, or a full skirt to camouflage heavy thighs. It may reveal your fabulous décolleté or thrill bystanders with a glimpse of your knees. It may dance over your chest, only to make a big play of your delightful waist. Only you will recognize when you have found your glory dress – you'll know from your smile as you introduce it to the mirror for the first time.

Discovering a cut which best suits your body requires both perseverance and ingenuity. Once you find it, clasp it to your grateful bosom and never let it go. Here are a few hints to get you going:

✳ **An A-line is a kind line**. This shape manages the diplomatic trick of making your shoulders appear less broad, while skating over the usual no-zones of belly, bum and thigh (BBT – that classic sandwich of little-loved body bits). It's what fashion writers are wont to call a no-brainer dress, because it marries form to function and you needn't give it a fig of thought.

✳ Shall I wrap that for you, madam? If you possess a substantial chest, this one's for you, escorting the eye down the inviting gulley of its plunge to arrive at a waist made all the more petite because of the structure above and the rippling skirt below. The seminal wrap, of course, came from Diane von Furstenberg way back in the seventies, when it ruled at Studio 54 and Park Avenue, doing D-I-S-C-O and generally causing a wicked stir. By the middle of that decade, DvF was turning out fifteen thousand dresses a week. As Von Furstenberg says: 'The wrap dress made women feel what they wanted to feel like . . . free and sexy . . . It also fitted in with the sexual revolution: a woman who chose to could be out of it in less than a minute!' It was liberation for women, and – vitally – it was also unexpectedly forgiving. 'What is so special about it,' DvF says of the dress she reintroduced in 1997, 'is that it's a very traditional form of clothing. It's like a toga, it's like a kimono, without buttons, without a zipper. What made my wrap dresses different was that they were made out of jersey and they sculpted the body.' Aha! Sculpted. That's the key – and until you've given one a spin, you won't truly understand its benevolent blessings, the way it fires up a figure, ignores a bulge and is uncommonly kind to a waist when trousers feel that bit too tight. 'I would say the wrap dress is better when you are a bit curvier,' says its inventor. Go buy!

✳ The empire, on which the sun never sets. If, like me, you have a pushy belly, then the empire line will love you. It's obvious why – that just-below-the-breast seam allows any kind of malarkey to be hidden by the looser fabric below. Breathe easy. Diet Dress to the rescue.

✳ Drop your waist, drop a dress size. If you are thick in the middle – and, darlings, we know who we are – then the simple expedient of a dropped waist will achieve much the same effect as an empire line, tricking the eye away from your belly, in this case allowing attention to rest, comfortably, on your hip. The hip is a mighty fine place to rest – as women who adore low-waist jeans will testify: the body is stretched, the bottom shrinks, the woman inside shines like a sunbeam and rocks the room.

✳ If in doubt, get Lucky (or Galaxy, or Power . . .). There's usually a dress of the season, and by some genius law of fashion physics, it is generally a Diet Dress. Thus, Roland Mouret's Galaxy dress a while back was the absolute masterclass in the art. It held you in, pushed you up and sprang that trick of turning something loose and spongy (your BBT) into something altogether more taut and tantalizing. It did this by the mere expedient of its cut: its figure-framing capped sleeves, its sinuous zip from nape to hem, its darted, engineered fabric carved to flick and furl about the body like a shower of kisses.

More recently, you may have noticed the Lucky dress from Issa's designer Daniella Helayel, as seen on Scarlett Johansson, Hilary Swank, Kristin Davis and Kate Middleton. The fashion world is unanimous: this is a high-performance dress virtually guaranteed to make you feel brilliant. How? 'I think the Lucky is such a hit because it flatters every body shape,' says Helayel. 'I started designing dresses because I couldn't find any that suited my own body – I'm Brazilian and curvy. It just seems to be one of those dresses that everyone feels good in.' The square neckline flatters most busts, the stitched bodice is a torso-tamer, the full skirt gives the welcome impression of slim legs, slim waist, slim you (while coasting considerately over your butt). Alternatively, the Preen Power Dress – a regular in the label's collections – will do something similar with a bit more slice and a lot more va-va-voom. 'We set out for it to be the ultimate cocktail dress that pulls you in and gives you body confidence,' says Preen's designer Justin Thornton. The illusion is achieved in several cunning ways: wide straps slim the shoulder (and, crucially, allow you to wear a bra); tucks and pleats of high-tensile elastane swerve about the body, pumping up assets and navigating trouble spots; the tube skirt (which pulls everything in like a dog herding sheep) is softened by a second tier – so you don't look like a waitress in a girly bar; the whole edifice is lined with a second skin of 'Power Net', a tough contouring mesh used in corsetry. Holy smoke.

WHY A DRESS?

There's always a 'piece' that distils a season, a garment which will whisk you from last month to next in a mere wink of the eye. If you inhabit the right sort of places, you might occasionally find fashion folk in huddles, perhaps on swish banquettes, saying things like 'It's all about the cardigan!' or 'Pants! Fenestra, we're going big on pants!' This season it may be tulip skirts, next it could be pedal-pushers or pea coats. But usually, usually it's a dress, the undisputed stalwart of style. The reason for its towering popularity lies in its versatility, dress-up-ability, femininity and – crucially – the fact that you chuck it over your head and you're done. As designer Alber Elbaz of Lanvin puts it, 'What I love about the dress isn't just the prettiness and romance, but also the simplicity. I love the zip-in and zip-out. It's the most modern uniform.'

42 FIND THE RIGHT JEANS

I seem to be surrounded by perfect bottoms. Everywhere I turn, there's another one – getting into a cab, easing itself on to a bar stool, running up that hill. Over the years, I have become something of an expert in the derrière department, like one of those builders who can give a bottom marks out of ten, even while trowelling mortar on to breeze-blocks and eating a fried-egg bap. I take great interest in other girls' bottoms in the same way as I'm fascinated by their kitchens (if they're fabulous) and their relationships (if they're not). It's a hobby founded on envy, of course, but finessed by the thought that, with a little effort and a lot of abstinence, I too could have a bottom that behaves impeccably in a bikini.

The best behind I know belongs to my friend Freya, and it is always housed in a pair of red-hot jeans. Hot jeans have the right label (True Religion, Sass & Bide, Citizen of Humanity, Hudson, J Brand), in the same way that naff jeans don't. But here's the thing. It was only when I went on holiday with Freya and her super-bum that I realized it was *all* in the jeans. Her bottom was pretty average when let loose, so to speak. It was those jeans that made hers a butt worth watching.

Yup, nothing on earth can cup and cradle your assets so effectively as the perfect pair of jeans. 'They are,' says Mary Quant, 'the greatest invention ever.' But the question is how to lay your hands on that elusive beast, the perfect pair? As with most matters of style, it depends a lot on what you've got; a pear cannot hope to be a peach using jean therapy alone. But you can maximize your assets. Here's how:

✳ **Try, try, try**, then, when you find perfection, buy, buy, buy.

✳ **Generally speaking, big bottoms look smaller in a man's-cut jean** – invariably, they'll have a shorter 'top block', the distance between crotch and waistband, which minimizes the area covered. Hipsters have a similarly illusory effect.

✳ **Denim has immense tummy-flattening capabilities**. Says Katharine Hamnett, 'There's an element of corsetry in jeans cutting – it's tough enough to hold you in.' A flat-lying waistband sitting just below the navel is generally the most flattering – though it depends entirely on the contours of your body. If you need to tame a tummy, a higher waist will keep everything in line, restrained by all that glorious, dependable denim. Wear a longer top if you need to, to mask the magic.

✳ Women's jeans are traditionally tapered below the knee and roomier at the thigh, which tends to shorten and add bulk to a figure. Instead, **choose a straight-leg jean**, though I strongly support resurrecting the trend for boot-cut jeans, the most flattering fashion ever bestowed on womankind, with their implicit guarantee to elongate the leg and shrink a bottom.

What more, really, could you ask of a pair of jeans? Keep them lean at the thigh, with a sharp shoot of a kick from knee to hem.

✳ **Buy a size that sits comfortably** rather than one that clings to your thighs like a child on his first day at nursery.

✳ **Buy them long and wear heels.** Adding height is, of course, the most obvious way to look leggy if you're not. To diminish the tarty overtone, wear a heeled boot. Only original stitching looks acceptable at your hem, so buy one pair of jeans for flats and another for heels.

✳ If you have thighs of a certain size – I'm not pointing, I'm just saying – **beware jeans with those jazzy bleached or distressed zones** on the leg which will simply draw attention to the blights in your life.

✳ If you're seventeen and built like a sapling, go for bleached. Otherwise, **buy dark indigo: it is most forgiving.**

✳ Whatever you buy, **pay close attention to the back pockets,** which will alter the dimensions of a bottom by leading the eye in a certain direction: Levi's masterstroke on its timeless 501s was to add stitching in a V-shape, giving the illusion of a smaller, neater rump. Surely every girl's dearest, deepest wish?

✳ If you have a Houdini belly (one that's forever trying to escape), **take a look at Tummy Tuck Jeans** from US brand Not Your Daughter's Jeans. They feature a high Lycra content and a patented criss-cross panel designed to firm up your upholstery. Get them at notyourdaughtersjeans.com.

✳ **Once you've bagged your dream jeans, wear them often.** Wear them as a statement of style, not as a bored basic. Better still, wear your skinniest, tightest pair, particularly if you're feeling fat (do this at home if you can't face the public) – nothing will do more to put you off that piece of pie.

43 CHOOSE FIT CLOTHES, NOT FAT CLOTHES

Never wear a shapeless sweater in the hope that it will hide a multitude of sins; it won't. What you need are properly fitted clothes, tight to the torso, fitted to your figure. This is the most flattering and slimming silhouette for any body shape, and you will benefit from it in an instant. If you can afford to, ditch your budget habit (cheap often means clunky) and invest in fewer, more tailored, more expensive clothes. Don't be afraid to have garments altered to your specifications and measurements – not too tight, but just right – even if you bought them off the peg in a high-street chain. These Goldilocks clothes will shave off pounds, not ounces. Rather brilliantly, tailoring is one of the few fashion concepts that looks better as you age. It won't give you the time of day until you're thirty-three, and then it's all over you like an expensive suit. It is simply one of those good things that comes to those who wait – and, as many a former model will tell you, a great tailor will do *far* more for you than a great surgeon.

If in doubt (and not yet in debt), my strong advice is to reach for couturier Antony Price. The man who dressed Roxy Music, Duran Duran, Jerry Hall, Princess Diana and every glittery Glamazon in between is known in certain postcodes as 'the doctor'. His forte, based on decades of finessing and refinement, is illusion (he once designed high-waist trousers with curious seams running up the rear and called them 'arse pants' – and somehow you know what he means). 'I'm the man who has spent forty years measuring and studying women's bodies,' Price says. 'Not just thin women. Everyday real women. Real bosoms. Real problems. Women who have no tits and want them, and women who want them smaller. I *build* frocks.'

The bottom line, he says, is that 'shapely women look better in fitted clothes. If you have material hanging, you just look like a salad bowl with drooping lettuce. Corsetry enables you to take the fabric of the dress and bang it right against your skin where you immediately lose a size or two. Smooth, no bits or lumps.' Just what the doctor ordered, right?

Of course, all this comes at a price. But there are high-street chains that have picked up on our need for tucking, tricking and tailoring: look at Topshop, where designers Christopher Kane and Marios Schwab continue the Price tradition of asset management with their high-stretch, high-strength collections. The people at Karen Millen also know how to pour structure into an outfit. Your challenge is to step up, and step out in the cling. Let the fabric take the strain.

44 UNDERSTAND THE VALUE OF PERFECT BLACK TROUSERS

Work unstintingly until you discover a pair which flatter you. Buy three pairs. Keep them pristine, dry-cleaned and pressed, not in a jumbled heap on the floor. Why? Because they are the most forgiving, the most friendly, the most fantastic garment ever to stalk the face of the earth. Now, I know they don't seem like much, hanging there on the rail, minding their own business. I can almost feel your disappointment. But bear with me. Black trousers are my desert island garment. They can save the hour, the day, the outfit. They can take you to work and then escort you to the movies, then on to cocktails, dinner and home to flump in front of the TV. They'll get along with anything – a tee, a tux, a tissue-silk top scattered with seed pearls and silver sequins; they'll meet any colour head on and make it sing. They're versatile and vivacious, comfortable and cool. They're the sartorial equivalent of that lovely boyfriend your mum liked but you thought was too safe; and, like him, you never knew what you had till they were gone. Safe, perhaps. But my word, they're handsome.

Make sure, then, that they're not overly trend-led. I have one fabulous pair of blacks which are wide-legged, high-waisted, with turn-ups and a whole heap of swaggering attitude. Fine for high days when you want people to say, 'Wow, get those pants!' But the perfect pair simply needs to keep quiet and get on with the job in hand. Go for a simple straight leg and a fit that suits the quirks and kinks of your own figure. This means – yes – you need to try and try again. I find a flat-front with a knife-edge crease works best for me, but you may prefer a peg or a boot-cut or a low-slung waist. You will also need to think weight. Not yours, but theirs; have several pairs to cover all eventualities and weather conditions. I suggest the following as a short-cut to sartorial bliss:

✶ **Black wool suit trousers**. Not synthetic, not heavy-ply, not too try-hard, the kind of trousers you barely know are there, like the quiet kid at school who goes on to win the Nobel Prize for physics.

✶ **Black denim jeans**. Workaday stuff, sure, but almost immune to stains and scuffs, and therefore a wardrobe winner every time. Will labour hard on your behalf, working day and night shifts, back-to-back if necessary.

✶ **Black cotton Capris**. Wear with a broderie anglaise top, or a loose linen shirt, and you've got summer in the city sussed.

✶ **Black velvet jeans**. A garment that will party till dawn and then get up and take the kids to school.

✶ **Black satin trousers**. Just so chic.

TO CUT A LONG STORY SHORT

Your trouser hem ought to sit comfortably on the top arch of your foot, mid-vamp, like a battalion on the brow of a hill. Unless your desert island trousers are designed to be worn cropped or trailing the floor like a lovelorn Ophelia, make sure the hem stops right there, having pulled off the twin tricks of making your legs look long and your feet look petite.

45 BE PARTICULAR ABOUT WHERE YOU SHOP

Getting dressed in the twenty-first century is, as we all know, a pretty haphazard affair, but it is made all the more complicated by our increasingly unruly bodies and the apparent reluctance of the design world to take the blindest bit of notice. While manufacturers insist on making clothes to fit the traditional hourglass shape, only 8 per cent of women are still built that way, according to a recent report from North Carolina State University. It's a bit like car manufacturers refusing to make anything but car-seat covers for fifties Corvettes: much of what's on the market simply doesn't fit.

Designer Katharine Hamnett – never one to toe the party line in fashion – has long been mightily aggravated by the issue. 'The fashion industry ignores the true size of women at its peril,' she warns. 'As to why they do, stupidity is the only reason I can think of. It is the result of adhering unthinkingly to a tradition.'

Daisy Lowe, model and muse, seems to have given the issue some thought and arrived at a canny conclusion: 'I love curvaciousness,' she says. 'Curvy girls are the sexiest girls. If clothes were built for curvier women, which is most of the population, one: people would look better; two: designers would sell more clothes, and three: they wouldn't have to use tiny anorexic models.' True enough. But until the fashion industry shakes itself from its stupor, the best way to find labels to love your shape is to clear a morning and book a session with a fashion adviser or personal shopper. There are undiscovered labels out there which will work for you, and a professional will be able to ferret them out before you can say 'Have you got that in chartreuse?' They know very well that clothes don't come in standard sizes, that one brand's 12 is another's 14; they understand the quirks of cut and fit that are characteristic of a particular label. There is great value in a little expert advice, just so long as you keep your eyes open and your plastic under strict control. Topshop, Debenhams and Lakeside Shopping Centre have a free personal-shopper service. The Trafford Centre in Manchester and Meadowhall in Sheffield both contain stores that provide personal shoppers. Then there's Liberty, Harrods, Harvey Nicks, Selfridges – all of them offer it, often for free, so use it. Why should the A-list hog all the personal services? Go grab a bit for yourself. I recommend first-rate undies and a bikini-line appointment before you embark on an encounter in the cubicle.

WHY APPLES AND PEARS ARE BANANAS

For some reason, it is currently fashionable to size up a body, judge it, label it – and then dress according to a template, as if commanded by Moses himself. All over the country, from Suffolk to Somerset, from the highlands to the low, it's Apples or Pears. I regularly hear from women trying in vain to ascertain their shape, as if labelling a body will somehow make it look better in a halter-neck maxi-dress. 'Am I a Spoon?' comes a plaintive email from Wolverhampton; 'I think I'm a Flowerpot,' writes Rita in Devon. 'Is this normal?' No Rita, it's not. It is ludicrous.

Pigeonholing our blameless bodies in this way somehow misses the point of getting dressed at all. Fashion, if you're living it and loving it, is an intimate and glorious thing. It thrives on personality and attitude, complexion and lifestyle; it is sparked by age, contained by budget, driven by dreams, and influenced by a whole lot of other things that have nothing to do with the size of your bottom in relation to the width of your hips. What works for one size 14 won't necessarily work for another; what looks delicious on one 'Spoon' will make another look like a Ladle. If style truly worked in this plodding, reductive way, we'd all dress like drones – neutered, neutralized and desperately dull at parties.

You are not an abstract shape, hanging there in the ether, untethered by temperament and taste. You are a person, and the most effective way of dressing depends largely on what makes you feel good. To ascertain your shape, then, don't look in a book. Let your clothing be your guide: your favourite jeans will tell you so much more than your scales – or those Apples and Pears – ever could.

129

46 BEWARE VANITY SIZING

It is possible that, many moons ago, the world's clothing manufacturers got together for a PowerPoint presentation entitled 'How to Keep your Customer Satisfied'. And right there at the top of the list in big neon capitals was this simple directive: LIE.

Stick a smaller size on bigger trousers! It really is so easy and so very appealing. Yes, but it's a honey trap, people, and you don't have to be a complete ditz to fall for it. Here's a little fairy tale to illustrate my point. One day, not so long ago, I discovered from the interior of a pair of jeans that I was a size 8. A size 8! That's a 6 in the States! As you might expect, I was thrilled to tiny little pieces, and bought two pairs before the shop assistant could draw breath. I have size-8 friends, of course – more associates, really – women who look so fabulous in shorts that you want to take yourself outside and jump off the kerb into the path of an oncoming ice-cream van. But now, here I was, a size 8! I would spread the good news, I'd yell it from the rooftops, there'd be rejoicing in the—

Hang on a second. These jeans were suspiciously roomy. I got them home, and found that they bore precisely the same dimensions as my old size 12s that I'd shoved to the back of my wardrobe. I'd been framed.

'Vanity sizing is all about making women feel thinner than they are,' Yasmin Sewell, fashion director at Browns boutique in London's South Molton Street, told *The Times*. 'We want to wear brands that flatter us. We also work with several celebrity stylists who practise vanity sizing to keep their A-list clients happy. They will cut out a size-14 label and sew in a size-10 label. It's the same thing.'

Now I don't give two hoots what size you happen to be, but the issue is that these vanity sizes bear no relation to how much space we actually take up in a minibus or a bath. And the truth is – steel yourselves – that women have been growing dramatically wider and heavier since the fifties, while the sizing we see on our labels has simply grown to accommodate our new girth. A recent UK

National Sizing Survey found that, over the last five decades, women have added an average of 2.5 inches around the hips and 6.5 inches on the waist. The average British woman now measures 39-34-41. If you have prided yourself on being a size 10 for the past thirty years, you will have grown by as much as five inches in the waist and bust. We may smirk to ourselves, as we climb into a size-10 skirt, that Marilyn Monroe was a size 16. Hah, we think, breathing in to get that zipper up, what a monumental fattie she was! Marilyn, for the record, had a 22-inch waist. In today's parlance, that makes her a pretty meagre size 8.

'Women have been growing dramatically wider and heavier since the fifties, while the sizing we see on our labels has simply grown to accommodate our new girth.'

Vanity sizing is now so widespread that a peculiar vacuum has emerged at the lower end of the spectrum as smaller sizes are commandeered for larger clothes, giving rise to the zeros and double-zeros that have so exercised the press of late. Any time now, we'll be into negative numbers, worn by women who are the shape and size of julienned vegetables. 'I'm a minus 4!' they'll chirrup from behind the changing-room curtain. 'By the laws of physics, I no longer exist!'

What this means for the humble punter – of any size – is that you can't trust a label, you *must* try it on. At M&S, for instance, a size 10 is significantly larger than a size 10 at Topshop, with its younger clientele. Miu Miu's 10s are notoriously minuscule (Brix

The psychology behind the practice is enough to make you rue the day you were born a woman. Apparently, 10 per cent of us cut the size tags out of our clothes so we don't have to see the number on a daily basis. Many of the rest of us prefer to live the lie, abetted by those cunning manufacturers who know that the smaller the size, the better we feel, ergo the more we'll buy.

Smith-Start, of Shoreditch designer boutique Start, told *The Times*, with admirable candour, that 'Designers size their clothes meanly because they want to keep big people out of them. Having fat people wear your clothes is not good for a brand's image. It's a fact of life.') The brute fact is that certain design houses simply don't want heavier people wearing their collections – perhaps because beautiful, slim-line people perpetuate the myth that only beautiful, slim-line people wear their clothes. With many top-end labels, as Smith-Start says, 'If you are curvy and have an arse – forget it.'

Clearly, different design houses and manufacturers have wildly opposing views of what makes a size 10, 14 or 18. I was once (briefly, years ago) the in-house model for Nicole Farhi, and they used my body as the template for a size 10 just because I happened to be hanging around doing the filing. It can be as random as that.

Little wonder, then, that 60 per cent of UK women admit to being unsure of their dress size. If you don't know your ins and outs, it's time to find out. You need clothes which *fit* rather than flatter to deceive, regardless of that pesky little number breathing down your neck and whispering velvet compliments in your ear. Shove yourself into clothes that are the wrong size and you'll very likely look fat. Or stupid. Possibly both. Ignore the numbers and concentrate on the look. That, after all, is what matters most.

STICK IT TO THE SIZEISTS

What to do about the boutiques which refuse to stock anything above a size 12? The designers who produce clothes only fit for mannequins? Boycott their handbags, people! Shame them by complaining loudly at the till. Write letters to *The Times*. Picket! I'm not expecting all labels to accommodate all sizes, but more availability for those of us who fall within the bell-curve of normal would be smashing, thanks ever so.

47 FIND *YOUR* SHOP

As Alexandra Shulman, editor of *Vogue*, once told me, 'It helps to
know the designers that suit you, to find your shop, so you're not
starting from scratch every time . . . Having some idea of your own
style, your strengths and weaknesses, helps – although, of course,
they do change as you get older. Personally, I find it much harder
to get away with boho dressing than I once did. You can so easily
look like an ageing Mystic Meg.'

Indeed. In my experience, one productive visit to a beloved
shop is worth a dozen schizophrenic trips along Bond Street in
desperate search of the New You. Leave that to Madonna's stylists,
and concentrate instead on a confidence-building, I-am-who-I-am
approach to shopping. Why do you think Kate Moss always
wears J Brand jeans? Why does Angelina Jolie swear by her Anya
Hindmarch bags? Why is Kate Middleton wedded to Issa? Not
because these women don't have all the choice in the world, but
because they have *made* a choice: they've found a faithful fashion
friend and they're not about to switch allegiance just because
the wind has changed direction.

Once you have found the place that works for you – it may be
a certain boutique, a particular designer, a chain-store which feels
like home – stick with it. Not religiously, but regularly. Don't be
too promiscuous. Personally, I have been so hooked on Gap for the
past decade that I get a bit antsy if I haven't rifled through the
rails from one month to the next. It works for me. It may not work
for you. Once you have discovered your shop, keep it close, keep it
constant, using it as a cornerstone of your look. Then throw curve
balls at it to pep things up and keep them guessing in the galleries.

48 BUY THE RIGHT SWIMSUIT

Every year, it happens. You look up from Easter and what do you know? Bikini time again. The most challenging weeks of your life are looming on the sun-kissed horizon, and you've just spent the last fortnight waist-deep in chocolate buttons. In your mind's eye, you're Ursula Andress emerging from the surf. You're Halle Berry in *Die Another Day*. You're Brigitte Bardot at Club 55. In reality, you're deluded, and you need all the help you can get, and fast. So, to all ye about to set sail for the shops to find that rare treasure, the bikini which will turn you into Scarlett Johansson with one ping of a Lycra-rich waistband . . . Well, here's the skinny, my friends.

✳ **There are classics in this game**, and no one should leave home during a hot spell without the reliable armour of a well-cut black one-piece. Stifle those yawns. Like the little black dress, this is the very backbone of a successful wardrobe, and without it, you'll merely wobble along on the very periphery of beach chic. If black feels dull, turn to your accessories to make the splash you want: a giant bag in a floral print, a pair of spangly flip-flops, even big wooden beads (not to be worn as you dive in the deep end or you'll knock yourself out).

✳ If you want your bikini to **work**, rather than simply take it easy on a lounger, you need to look for the following:

Underwiring, which will stop your breasts heading down Mexico way.

A top with clip fastenings, not ties: these will give you added stability and eliminate the exhausted flop of so many bad bikinis.

A tie-side bottom, though, is forgiving and won't bite into your rump like a wide-side tends to.

High-leg pants will elongate a leg, but also demand exhibition-class depilation.

When entering the sea, **do try not to fiddle with your bikini**. You look fine, really. Pulling fabric from between your cheeks won't improve matters one iota and may serve to make things worse.

✳ Better yet, **buy a Miracle Suit**. Having spent most of my life – or at least the beach-bound portion of it – wearing natty little bikinis in Aegean-blue, I recently discovered that I need a little helping hand if I am to look even the same *species* as a Kelly Brook or a Helen Mirren (a woman twenty years my senior who makes me want to bay at the moon in jealous anguish). Still, as Helen herself knows, at a certain age we all require a push here, a pick-up there. A bit of illusion. And this, dear reader, is where the Miracle Suit comes in. Tag line: 'Ten pounds lighter in ten seconds!' Way to go! The cut has a hint of the fifties about it, with a substantial bottom, an elegant swathe at the décolletage, and a tremendous capacity to contain, thanks to a fabric with several times the tensile strength of Lycra. As a result, it makes you walk like a screen goddess and look like a babe. Dynamite. All this comes at a cost (around £100, though less expensive versions are increasingly available). There's also the vaguely unsettling sense that you've waltzed back in time to an era when women were tied to the stove and bound by their formidable underwear. Still, what price beach pride, eh?

✳ Of course, you could always rest easy in the comforting embrace of a **beach kaftan**. It may not be the very pinnacle of cool, but there's no shame in it; this is easily one of the best fashion inventions of recent times, marrying as it does a nonchalant ethnicity with an unfussy chic. More to the point, it covers an entire catechism of sins and allows the wearer to feel, just for this short time, that they live on the same planet as Elizabeth Hurley. Bliss – not to mention a bonus for anyone who happens to be sitting behind you as you dive for the Frisbee on the soft white sand.

'If you want a bikini which will turn you into Scarlett Johansson with one ping of a Lycra-rich waistband ... Well, here's the skinny, my friends.'

49 RECOGNIZE THAT THERE ARE SOME CLOTHES YOU SHOULD NEVER WEAR

Leafing through the *New York Times* recently, I came across this pearl of sartorial wisdom: 'A leather belt works well over knits.' Oh really? Have you tried it? In the interests of research (I put the hours in for you, really I do), I buckled a wide leather belt at waist level over my old Cornish fisherman's sweater – and what did I look like? A roll of loft insulation. Bottom line: a leather belt *never* works well over knits, unless you are built like a broom handle, and even then your friends will very likely discuss behind your back how dumpy you've become.

Which got me thinking. While I have always been scrupulous with the truth when ruminating upon the intricacies of fashion, I am suspicious that my contemporaries out there are sometimes less than entirely honest. To put things straight, I have compiled the following checklist of Style Lies that you may want to cut out and keep, perhaps in your purse, to be pulled out when confronted with a pile of duplicitous glossy magazines at the hairdresser's.

✳ **It is not OK to wear a mini over the age of thirty-nine.** I am forty-one. Trust me. There is a cut-off point and this is it.

✳ Unless you are a MacDonald or a Campbell or a model for Burberry, **tartan is not the answer to winter dressing.**

✳ **Bags shaped like 'things' (toy dogs, flowerpots, threatened wildlife) are not clever.** They are idiotic. Get a chihuahua.

✳ **Ochre is not an 'It colour'.** Along with a host of other shades, it is very tough to wear, whatever Giorgio Armani would have us believe. I include on my list: tangerine (and, while we're at it, the entire orange family, which should be treated gingerly) and salmon (together with all of the mid-pinks, including Elastoplast, Pepto Bismol and ointment). Don't swallow a catwalk colour directive simply because it appears to come from on high (very often, these things are decided years in advance by a fabric focus group in a Geneva conference room). Your *own* colouring will determine the colours you wear most successfully. Find a palette that you adore and it will adore you in return. As my friend Tim says, it never hurts to ask if an item comes in another colour besides yellow.

✴ **You do not need a new handbag every season.** Sure, it would be nice, but weren't you saving up for a trip to Paris?

✴ **The only people who look good in capes are superheroes and Mary Poppins.** If you are not one of the above, leave well alone. Similarly, ponchos are for gauchos. Ditto chaps.

✴ **A Chanel jacket will not make you thin or beautiful.** But it will make you happy.

Armed with this useful list, you will now be able to scythe through the Style Lies that litter your life. You will feel free, fabulous and five pounds lighter. OK, that's a lie. But you might just stop putting leather belts over your sweaters. Small mercies, I say.

WHAT NOT TO WEAR:
A QUICKFIRE CHECKLIST

In the meantime, do bear in mind that there are some clothes that you should never wear if you want to walk on the skinny side. They include:

✴ Puffa jackets.

✴ Belted cardigans.

✴ Outsize knitwear.

✴ Your partner's jeans.

✴ Hot pants and boob tubes.

✴ Sweater dresses.

✴ Tweed in general. Layered tweed in particular.

✴ I'd also advise that you think v-e-r-y carefully about strapless (particularly on your wedding day). There are about twelve people on the planet who look truly brilliant in a strapless frock, and – love you as I do – it's unlikely that you're one of them. If in doubt, pull on a shrug.

137

50 NEVER BUY CLOTHES FOR THE WOMAN YOU'D LIKE TO BE, BUY THEM FOR THE WOMAN YOU ARE

We've all got them, haven't we? The Moroccan slippers. The leather trousers. The baby-doll dress, the trilby, the shortie-shorts that looked so great on Kate Moss at Glastonbury. All those items we bought for the life we'd *like* to have, rather than the one we're living. My world is thick with whim purchases for the woman I'll never be: the exfoliating thigh mitt (can't be bothered), the phone which plays music and takes photos (don't know which buttons to press), the white Chanel coat (way too beautiful to wear), the wetsuit (way too ugly to wear) . . .

Even such mavens of style as Sarah Jessica Parker suffer from this kind of displacement shopping. 'There are so many clothes I want,' she said in a recent interview. 'I want more gold cuffs, some great Fendi bags and anything Nicolas Ghesquière has done for Balenciaga. And of course I want shoes, shoes and more shoes . . . And the other thing I can't get enough of is vintage, vintage, vintage . . . But so much of this is for the woman I think I should be, but the woman I really am is, sadly, going less and less to the shops.'

My problem is that I have no problem *whatsoever* going to the shops. When I get there, though, I can quite easily convince myself that there is room in my life for another scarlet lipstick, even though it makes me look like a transvestite and I have never once worn it outside my own bathroom. The dream is, of course, what gets us out there, trying on a life and buying up a future, even if it's never going to fit. It's how all advertising works – we're sold the idea that we live in a beach house in New England, though it's quite clear that we're stuck in a semi in Stoke. And so we buy the wicker furniture that would indeed look great on a wraparound porch looking out over the ocean. We stuff it in the lounge and hope for the best. The danger is that we spend so much time indulging in a fantasy life, one where we're thinner, wittier, better at diving or chess, that we forget to live our own.

The key to dressing thin is knowing – seeing, believing – the state you're in. Thus there are things that I have ushered out of my life because they simply don't work for me. Those racer-backed tops which can't be worn with a bra? Hmm. If I don't wear a bra, I frighten small children. The plaid coat? Looks better as a picnic rug. The lovely polka-dot dress which would be a dream if only I didn't own quite such conversational breasts? Out, out damn spots! The point here is that you are not Sienna Miller. You are not Fearne Cotton. You are not Helena Christensen. You are you. Wonderful, glorious you.

51 DISCOVER WOMEN DESIGNERS

This won't make you fall off your stool in astonishment, but women designers are usually more accommodating of the female body, and therefore worth investigating if you want to give yours an advantage. Most of them admit to designing for their own figures – itself hardly surprising since that's the body they have to dress every day and the one that's closest to hand in the design studio. Betty Jackson's gentle designs, for example, work well for women who – like herself – want to look taller and slimmer. Donna Karan, one of my heroines and a woman who well knows the value of high-tensile Spandex, refuses to design clothes which can't be worn by a size 12 or 14 (and that's US sizing, which translates to a 14 or 16 in the UK, the kind of size which might make Julien Macdonald collapse on the floor in a frilly heap).

'I'm dealing with the fallibility of a woman's body,' Karan once told me. (We were at one of those parties which happen fairly often in fashion – for some reason best known to her publicity department, a vast Shepherd's Bush warehouse had been transformed for one night only into a sultan's pleasure-drome.

Or perhaps it was a Balinese palace. Either way, I remember rather a lot of scatter cushions.) 'My own shape is rounded,' she said, over the din of the twenty-four-piece Congolese drumming band. 'I don't have a perfect body . . . Show me a woman who does.' Karan apparently tests clothes on herself to eliminate gaping shirts and bulging contours and reputedly designs naked in front of the mirror. 'I share my secrets with other women,' she said recently. 'It's a communication of ways to delete the negative and accent the positive. Let's face it, we all want to look tall and thin.'

Katharine Hamnett, by contrast, started designing precisely because she *is* tall and thin: sleeves and trousers were always too short, making her look like an extra in *Oliver!* As Helen Storey – a great designer of the nineties – once put it, 'There are bits I can trust, bits I know are familiar to other women. Clothes made by women don't deny what's underneath – we dress the essence, not the male-inspired dream.'

So, with female designers you get no coned breasts, no steel corsets, no pussy pelmets. Not quite so many slut shoes. No bound feet or bustles (Rei Kawakubo and Vivienne Westwood being the exceptions that prove the rule). Women designers – from Stella McCartney to Nicole Farhi, from Vera Wang to Donatella Versace – tend to have known the burden of fat days, dark days, down days and frizzy-hair days. They know the aggravation of that impish squeeze of flesh which escapes a bra. They've probably tucked their skirt into their knickers on occasion or lost a heel to a sidewalk. While male designers can have imaginations that take them on a soaring journey of creativity, it tends to be the women who know what it feels like when a pencil skirt is cut too tight, recognizing that careful cutting, deft drapery and an eye on the bottom line are what it takes to dress a woman well. As Diane von Furstenberg, herself a dab hand at the support and tenderness required to properly furnish a figure, says, 'Personally, I have always been attracted to clothes designed by women. Coco Chanel, Vionnet, Norma Kamali, Donna Karan. They have a little more – how do I put it? – *understanding*.' Listen up, sisters. Listen and learn.

52 PRACTISE WARDROBE FENG SHUI

When I moved into my current house, I somehow scored a proper walk-in wardrobe. The sheer delight of *walking in*, pirouetting around and alighting on today's clever choice of shoe, shirt or shape-wear! You can see it now, can't you? Neat ranks of Manolos, lined up and ready to do battle on my behalf. A flight of colour-coordinated cashmere. Boxes of cross-referenced accessories, with an efficient Polaroid index of where and when they were last seen. Ironed pants. How dreamy.

And a dream it is. My friend Lucy stumbled into my 'walk-in' not so long ago and fell over a discarded mattress. 'Is there a light in here?' she hollered, in a muffled sort of voice which sounded like a small woman trapped under a large mattress. 'I think I've stubbed my chin. Is that a lawnmower?'

Lucy had entered the Pit, as this small room is fondly known, in search of a T-shirt to replace the one her first-born, Orlando, had just vomited over. Wrist-deep in tomato ketchup myself, and grappling with a child who wanted to post chips up his own nose, I had gaily waved her off in the general direction of my wardrobe and told her to take anything which came to hand.

What came to hand, it transpired, was an old bedspread, a set of wheely suitcases, a cup of cold coffee, an original Pucci scarf and my last Dyson but one. (Not a lawnmower. Even I am not that weird.)

Somehow, though, from beneath the chaos, I managed to collate an outfit each day, by pot-luck really. An old fashion hack once congratulated me on my inspired pairing of sailor's trousers and pussy-bow blouse – little knowing that, like all great works of art, it was but an accident of fate.

Now, though, Lucy was on to me. Oh, the shame. In certain circles, I am considered to know a thing or two about clothes. People turn to me for advice – like the woman who messaged me for help in locating a pair of 'elderberry-coloured shoes' to go with the table decorations at her sister's wedding. And yet I clearly

141

treated my own clothes with utter disrespect. Shirts were shucked off and left on the floor, in the dark, neglected overnight. I had single earrings, whose partners had left the building in search of a more sympathetic home. I once moved a stepladder to one side and discovered my black Gucci dress attached to one of its rubber feet. I'd been looking for it for months, and had secretly put Violetta, our Ukrainian cleaner, in the frame.

And I knew I wasn't alone. Surely, I said to Lucy, the only people with neatly folded clothes are obsessive compulsives, bored housewives, gay men and people who work in Benetton? 'No,' she retorted tartly. 'You are a wardrobe tramp. You need to feng shui the lot, like Elton John and Boy George do every so often. It will give you inner peace.' And more space for new shoes! I liked the way she thought.

And so, with Lucy in mind, I undertook a wholesale reorganization of the Pit. It took hour upon committed hour, thanks to the sheer mountain of guff I'd managed to accumulate even while attempting to live a frugal, eco-conscious, streamlined life. Take gloves. I had five pairs of evening gloves, two pairs of driving gloves, fifteen pairs of woolly gloves, two pairs of snowboarding gloves and a pair of Sasquatch furry mittens from Yohji Yamamoto. I also had twelve pairs of trainers, plus a pair of ballooning loon pants in orange viscose. I still owned a beloved red cashmere sweater that died years ago, tragically, in a hot wash, and a half-made skirt given to me by Alexander McQueen before he got famous. At the backest back of my wardrobe, I discovered six pillows which *I had never seen before*. How could this be?

It wasn't just quantity, though. The whole process of slimming down my wardrobe took for ever because I'm a sentimental old fool. Every article trawled from its depths had its own story, its own tale to tell. Here were the zebra-print Dior mules which walked through Hyde Park in the pouring rain and lost a heel on Horse Guards Parade. Here was the vintage forties tea-dress which I wore, invariably, for four months of 1998; I couldn't live without it, until a new model came along and stole my heart. And there was the hot-pink mohair sweater which I stopped wearing the day I heard

P. J. O'Rourke's compelling comment on women's clothes ('Never wear anything that panics the cat').

The funny thing is how tender one feels about past outfits, even though we allow them to lie unloved in the closet, eclipsed by snazzier, sassier replacements. Even now, the smell of my ancient denim jacket – the one that took me to Mexico and rode horses on the beach at Cabo San Lucas, the one that met my husband on the same day as I did, the one that was lost for a whole week and turned up in lost property at St Pancras – is a Proustian fix. Its warm, comforting tang is my history, its texture my past.

'I once moved a stepladder to one side and discovered my black Gucci dress attached to one of its rubber feet.'

This, however, is no time to play Misty. A wardrobe needs to work – hard – in your defence. So get to it. Throw out clothes which no longer fit. Chuck out items which carry a hint of Agnetha Fältskog or early Spandau Ballet. Rid yourself of anything you haven't worn for two years, no matter how painful the parting. I suggest you axe the stone-wash denim, the fake-fur muffler and anything, however inoffensive, in corduroy. If it's vintage Galliano, stick it on eBay and reinvest.

Since my fashion feng shui, I can report that life has become a sight more simple. Just having the right clothes available at the right time – a great sweater here, a top top there, pressed and not pummelled to pieces, a blouse that you haven't seen for years but which works the tush off those cigarette pants – well, it makes dressing a breeze. The consequence is a more considered look. The consequence of this in turn is a better-dressed you. The consequence of this? Guess what: you've just lost weight.

53 DRESS YOUR AGE, NOT YOUR SHOE SIZE

OK, my feet happen to be a thirty-nine so the aphorism doesn't quite work. However, the point is that we should really entertain more realistic style crushes as the clock ticks on. It's fine to dress like Agyness Deyn, Peaches Geldof or Mary-Kate Olsen if you still live in the box room with your menagerie of cuddly toys. But the rest of us would do well to look beyond their tiddly skirts, kooky capes, hand-span T-shirts and minuscule fur jerkins, without sacrificing a sense of informed, inspired style.

While fashion pundits tend to be terribly gung-ho about the agelessness of clothes, about how the taboos of dress have been broken, and how mother and daughter can now wear the same outfit to the same party where they'll dance to the same song around the same handbag, the truth is that there *are* still boundaries. Not, perhaps, enforced by a culture of strictures and codes, but by the fact that a forty-year-old woman wearing lamé culottes looks plain daft. Youthful clothes tend to revel in the fizzy fact that they are cheap and cheerful, which necessarily means that not a great deal of thought has been lavished on navigating a rounded tummy or catering for heavier breasts.

While mid-lifers are struggling with the mirror, though, the fashion world remains haughtily besotted with youth, enthralled by its milk skin and pretty feet. For the time being – at least until the fashion industry wakes up to this mature market hungry to spend money on clothes – it's up to you to dress appropriately. Know thyself (you should already be halfway there) – and that elusive word 'style' will start to follow you around like a puff of Chanel No 5. For a lesson in how to go about it, over to Carine Roitfeld, the fifty-something editor of French *Vogue*. Her look – punch-black eyes and a wall of hair which threatens to close off her face from public view – is imitated everywhere: on the catwalk, in the ad pages of the glossies, in the windows of department stores. 'Right now,' said a recent paean, 'Carine Roitfeld is the most stylish woman in the world.'

So, Carine? How's it done?

'Leather trousers?' she says firmly. 'No good as you get older . . .
For normal woman, with not big money, if I would give advice:
buy mainly classic pieces and a new pair of shoes each season.
A Burberry trench-coat is always beautiful. Maybe you change
the belt and this season you put an Indian scarf.' Little things.
Big difference. Proper clothes. Slimmer you.

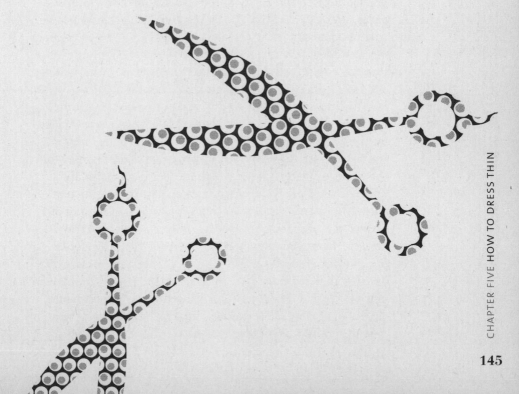

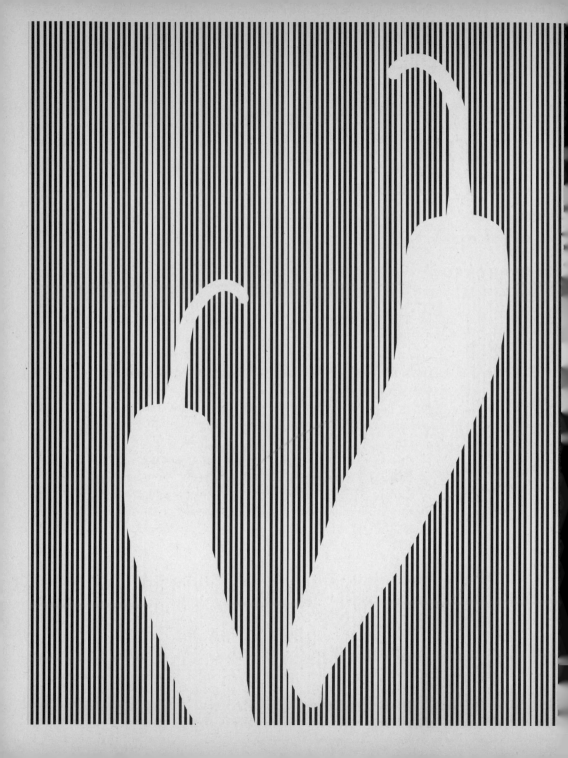

CHAPTER SIX
HOW TO EAT
PETITE
Part 2: Master the Art of Calorie Killing

As you will by now have registered, this is not a diet, it's a live-it, all about simple methods which modify your behaviour to maximize your chances of looking knockout in that little black dress. I'm not about to demand that you ban the butties, but the truth is that some fun foods just aren't worth the calories. Banish the ones you don't adore, the ones you could take or leave, and only eat because they happen to be sitting in front of you on a nice big plate. Regard the others as special-occasion treats and afford them respect, like a visiting dignitary. This chapter examines the what, why and how of effort-free calorie-slaying. There's masses of meat on this particular bone, so rather than feeling overwhelmed by the smorgasbord of choice, cherry-pick what works for you, remembering all the while that this is about enjoyment not torment. It should feel as easy as taking candy from a baby.

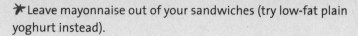

54 PRACTISE CALORIE SKIMMING BY ELIMINATING THE EASY THINGS

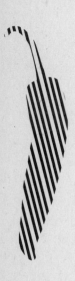

✳ Leave mayonnaise out of your sandwiches (try low-fat plain yoghurt instead).

✳ Lose the sugar in your tea.

✳ Have sorbet instead of ice-cream.

✳ And a dunk of olive oil rather than butter.

✳ Change full-fat to skimmed.

✳ Go from white to wholemeal.

✳ Order spritzer not wine.

See? You'll hardly notice the difference, but your buttocks will.

Here's more:

✳ Serve crudités not crisps when friends come for drinks.

✳ If eating out at a decent restaurant, ask for carrot sticks not grissini (if in New York, phone ahead and book 'em).

✳ Give the bread basket the cold shoulder.

✳ Ditch the ketchup. More than 120 million bottles are sold every year in the UK, but it is sugary condiments like this that clock up the calories; if you need sauce, make your own salsa with finely chopped tomatoes, spring onions and a hit of chilli.

✳ Choose fish over meat. And grill your fish, don't batter it.

✳ Similarly, skin your chicken, trim the fat off your meat and never eat pork crackling again, remembering that it is a pig's epidermis and not a delicious and entertaining treat.

✳ If you must eat beef or lamb, choose 'grass-fed' or 'pasture-raised' meat: it has significantly less fat, fewer calories and more Omega 3s than grain-fed meat (and also implies that the animal was humanely raised).

✴ Extend your meat-eating to include lean game. Venison, for example, has just 10 per cent of the fat found in beef.

✴ Keep frozen bananas, frozen blueberries, homemade fruit-juice lollies or granita in the freezer instead of ice-cream.

✴ Buy tuna in brine; try sun-dried tomatoes which are *dried*, not bathing in oil.

✴ Use non-stick spray-on oil in your (seldom-used) frying pan.

✴ Graduate from beef to turkey.

✴ Have a cheese holiday (that's time-out from cheese, not a weekend break in Leicester).

✴ Go from lattes to Americanos, cappuccinos to black filter. If you're a milk monster, just go skinny.

✴ Sacrifice caffeine altogether if you can, since it is considered to make the body acidic, which encourages the accretion of fat. Develop a green-tea habit instead (see below).

✴ Favour mushrooms over meat: a study at John Hopkins Weight Management Center has come to the remarkable conclusion that eating meals made of mushrooms – lasagne, chilli, whatever – rather than lean ground beef results in fewer calories being consumed at each meal. The difference averaged 420 calories and 30 grams of fat per day. Another study found that if men substituted a four-ounce portabella mushroom for a four-ounce grilled hamburger every time they ate a burger over the course of a year, and didn't change anything else, they could save more than 18,000 calories and nearly 3,000 grams of fat, the equivalent of 5.3 pounds or 30 sticks of butter. That is a heck of a lot of fat (but, one can't help noticing, quite a lot of mushrooms too; perhaps take a modest approach and make an occasional swap).

✴ Choose fresh fruit over dried: the drying process concentrates both nutrients *and* calories – which is all very well if you're hiking in the High Andes and haven't got much room in your rucksack.

But on an average day, choose fresh. A cup of fresh apricots, for instance, has around 74 calories and more vitamin C than a cup of the dried fruit, which clocks up three times the calories.

✳ Buy only 80 per cent cocoa-solids chocolate. Better still, sleep through Easter and Christmas (or get religion and do Lent).

✳ Do research so you know what you're putting into your system. Only 5 per cent of people in Starbucks, and 3 per cent in McDonald's, bother to read the nutritional leaflets on offer – but it's an easy way to arm yourself with knowledge and make informed swaps. So, in Wagamama, for instance, don't choose Yaki Udon (udon noodles with shiitake mushrooms, prawns, chicken, kitchen sink: 701 calories); choose Seafood Ramen (noodle soup with grilled fish and tiger prawns: 190 calories). Starbucks' passion cake, meanwhile, is 528 calories a slice; its lemon drizzle cake is 198 …

DRINK YOURSELF THIN WITH GREEN TEA

I well remember the first time I saw Sophie Dahl, years ago, rolling down a catwalk, all thigh and breast and come on, barely contained in a cobweb of angora on the catwalk of Irish designer Lainey Keogh. Compared to most of the girls who rattled down the runway, Dahl was vast, a glorious confection of marshmallow, peaches and cream. We fashion editors loved it, Sophie found fame fast, and then – as if by magic – she shed two stone, seven pounds and three dress sizes. While will-power must have played a strong hand, Sophie herself name-checks the invigorating, fat-busting power of green tea. 'I slimmed from a size 16 to a 12 by sipping cups of green tea, which helps to speed up the metabolism,' she said at the time of her incredible shrink. This elixir has been hailed as a cancer-fighter, an allergy-slayer, a heart-protector – but all you really need to absorb for our present purposes is that it has virtually no calories, and about half the caffeine of coffee. The same goes for ancient Chinese Pu-er tea, a favourite of Joss Stone, Jerry Hall and Victoria Beckham. It comes in cake form and needs to be crumbled into boiling water, with a view to raising the metabolism without stressing the heart. This clever concoction apparently burns extra calories without one having to lift so much as a thumb, which means that women – *thin* women – speak in hushed and grateful tones of its capacity to melt fat and reduce cholesterol. But, hey, you don't even need to buy the hype. Just know that a milk-free tea is your drink of choice should you want to shift some baggage.

If you need a little persuasion to tear yourself away from the cappuccinos you're addicted to, consider the *Which?* report of January 2008 which found that coffee from high-street chains can contain hundreds *and hundreds* of calories per cup. Don't get mugged by a fattuccino; it's time to wake up and smell the calories (you'll save a fortune too):

✳ Starbucks venti white-chocolate whole-milk mocha with whipped cream, **628 calories** (nearly a *third* of your total recommended daily calorie allowance).

✳ Caffè Nero medium semi-skimmed mocha with whipped cream, **326 calories**.

✳ Costa mocha medio whole-milk flake, **297 calories**.

✳ Costa caffe latte medio with full-fat milk, **123 calories**.

✳ Costa caffe latte medio with skimmed milk, **71 calories**.

✳ Starbucks double espresso, **11 tiny little calories**.

55 TAKE THE FOOD FACTOR OUT OF THE EQUATION

As Stephen Fry put it with such perspicacity, 'How did I lose the weight? Prepare to be astonished – I ate less food. That is the only way.' There are, however, ways to consume less *and not even notice*. This is the key to non-diet weight loss, the clever way to slim down naturally, effectively, sustainably, healthily and (crucial, this) enjoyably, particularly in a culture where food is everywhere you look, waiting to trip you up and get you face-down in a pecan pie.

Each day, we apparently make more than 250 food decisions. That means we have *choices*. So make the right ones. This applies to all food, whether it's from Le Gavroche or Le Greasy Spoon. Here's how:

✳ **Have business lunches in the office or in a park**, not in restaurants with four types of artisan bread and a tempting and comprehensive pudding menu.

✳ **Cut down on restaurant visits in general**, since you inevitably eat more when dining out (an average of 1,000 calories per meal, and that's not including the platter of nougat and macaroons that you will demolish by accident while waiting to pay the bill). I'm not suggesting you only ever eat at home, by the meagre light of a tallow candle. But do think twice before you climb into the car and rock up at Pizza Express.

✳ **If you are eating out, do a Bruce Willis**: when the star pops into the Ivy he asks the chef to steam his organic veggies. You may never have saved the world from certain Armageddon, but you too can be a bit of a diva in restaurants. This is the twenty-first century, people, so don't order what they give you, order what you want, and make it lite.

✳ **Ask for sauces on the side**, in a neat jug, not corrupting your plate with a puddle of superfluous calories. Do the same with dressing: request naked leaves and dress them yourself (with oil, vinegar, lemon, not blue cheese).

✱ **Say 'No dessert, thank you'** to the waiter *before* he offers you a list which includes sticky toffee pudding, treacle tart, chocolate fondant and three flavours of bespoke ice-cream. I mean, really, who wouldn't crumble?

✱ **Squeeze washing-up liquid on leftovers from the kids' tea**. I'm serious – if this is your vice, then slay it now. If a cold fishfinger is beyond resistance, then put it beyond temptation. Make whatever is left on the plate unavailable to nibble on, whether it's a napkin across the food, or, in another radical move, pouring salt over provocative leftovers. It may sound drastic, but it's the picking and the pecking that really piles on the pounds – ask any mother who suddenly has to cope with a whole new meal at teatime. Pretty soon, there's a whole new her in the mirror. As US comic Janette Barber says, 'When I buy cookies I eat just four and throw the rest away. But first I spray them with Raid so I won't dig them out of the garbage later. Be careful, though, because that Raid really doesn't taste that bad.'

✱ **Wrap tempting titbits in silver foil**, so they can't make eyes at you through a window of cling film. There's nothing like a leftover chicken drumstick for looking lonely and in need of rescue.

✱ **Kiss cook's perks goodbye** – whether it's the snatched crusts off your children's packed-lunch sandwiches, the 'tester' scone warm from the oven or cake mix straight from the bowl. This last – despite being an unpromising combination of raw egg and uncooked flour – remains one of the most delicious edibles I know. Buy a spatula. Scrape it all into the baking tin, not into your waiting maw.

✱ **If you happen to be in a self-service restaurant, don't use a tray**. Studies have shown that you are likely to fill it up, simply because it's there; only take what you can politely carry in your hands (stacking under your chin is not part of the deal). In fact, trays are fast being removed from college restaurants across the States in an effort to tackle obesity and cut food waste.

✳ Studies have also shown that if there are lots of options on offer at a buffet, you'll eat more. So **only put three things on your plate at a time**.

✳ OK, so now we're in the realms of mild excess, but if you're an incorrigible dough-head, you need to take action. When the waiter brings bread to the table, spill a glass of water on it. There. Out of bounds. Better still, more polite and infinitely more ethical, ask nicely for **'No bread'**, graduating to 'No poppadoms, no mayo, no whipped cream, no cocoa-dusted truffles and certainly no After Eights'. When dining out, then, only eat things that are specified on the menu, not all the feel-good freebie bonus bits which will propel you helplessly on to the plus side.

✳ **At home, serve vegetables and salad in heaped, welcoming, help-yourself bowls on the dining table**. Americans call this 'family style', which is nice. It makes me think of the Waltons and gives me a strong urge to bake a blueberry pie.

✳ **Keep meat, sausages, mashed potatoes, Yorkshire puddings and other fatteners back in the kitchen**, out of sight. Serve them on to individual plates.

✳ **Go food shopping after lunch**, not before. A standard supermarket easily becomes a grotto of gastronomic delights if you're starving, thanks to your hunger hormones. I have been known to fall heavily for Mr Kipling jam tarts – which, in truth, are vile – simply because I hadn't seen a calorie since breakfast. Go after lunch and you'll be far more circumspect in your purchases. Take PMT into any store, btw, and you'll come out with chocolate.

✳ **If you *do* come out with chocolate, break off two squares and put the rest away**, repeating to yourself: 'Nothing tastes as good as being thin feels' in a voice like Dorothy in *The Wizard of Oz*. Beware, then, the Proximity Principle: a study conducted at the University of Illinois (using Hershey's Kisses) showed how having food conveniently close makes you eat a whole lot more of it. When workers kept the chocolate on their desk, they ate an average of nine Kisses per day; when it was moved just six feet away, they ate only four per day. This is your cue to remove temptation. Don't give yourself the choice of whether to eat the nachos or not; don't put the nachos on the table. Better still, don't buy the nachos.

✱ **Similarly, keep sugar in a bag**, closed with a peg, housed in a Tupperware container with KEEP OUT stencilled on the top in biro. In the shed. Don't have it in a bowl, placed at a convenient distance from your elbow.

✱ **Just cook *enough*.** Not too much, but enough. Being of Italian descent, I generally boil twice the amount of pasta recommended on the packet, in the belief that too much is eminently and always preferable to too little. I invariably end up with great steaming vats of farfalle, pans brimming with fusilli, linguine as far as the eye can see. I then compensate for my profligacy by subjecting the plates to overfill. Pasta slips, slops and spills over the edges and quite often on to the floor, all voluptuous and glossy and fetching. I proceed to eat as much as I can (no, no, not off the floor), like one of those hicks from the sticks in a chilli-dog-eating contest. *Disaster.* The way to navigate this calorie pit is to avoid it completely. Cook less. An average portion of rice for an adult is 50g; for pasta it's 100g. You won't have to mop the floor so often either, so it really is win-win.

✱ **Be the last at the table to start eating**. And the first to stop.

✱ **Remember that leftovers are all the more delicious (somehow) for being surplus to requirements**. This is an oddity of food: it is so much more appealing when it's not on your plate but elsewhere (on your partner's plate, say). The gooey deliciousness that lurks under a warm roast chicken needs no introduction from me – and while it should perhaps remain in your world as an occasional treat, on the whole, try to strike the leftovers before they coo and woo. Either produce the right amount of food in the first place, or ditch any extra directly after serving. A cooling roast potato while you're drying the pots is a dangerous thing indeed.

CAKE FEAR:
LEARN TO LOATHE THE ONE YOU LOVE

Food, alas, is everywhere. We live in a food soup. And very seductive it is too. 'Food,' says Philip Hodson, fellow of the British Association for Counselling and Psychotherapy, 'is art, it's decoration, it's interior design. Humans have always used food symbolically, whether in ritual or religion – but now we tend to use it as a drug. It's a love substitute, a sex substitute. If you are touch-hungry, hungry for gratification, eating does, briefly, fill the void. The reason it's difficult to stop eating certain foods is that we're made to feel deprived of what is socially defined as a sensual pleasure.'

Remember, then, that food is only and always ephemeral. 'It is also,' says Hodson, 'anonymous: you can love it but it won't love you back.' Food is not a solution. It's a means, not an end. So it's time to demote. And, perhaps, time to end a few passionate relationships.

Personally – and I'll admit it's a weird talent – I can spot a slice of lemon drizzle cake across a crowded room. It is a rare meringue that gets past my eagle eye, particularly if it's laden with whipped cream and perhaps a lone strawberry. Chocolate cake actually talks to me, whispering sweet fudgy nothings from under its plastic dome, egging me on, closer, closer, until – *kaboom* – I'm staring at the empty, crumby plate wondering where it all went wrong and whether it would be beyond the pale to have another slice. Yup, we all have our soft spots. Winnie the Pooh's was honey. Popeye's was spinach. And mine is proper old-time teatime cake. Yours might be cheesy chips or Amaretto or those chocolate puddings that are gooey in the centre, as if they have recently fallen in love. Whatever it is, know it. Note it. Now destroy it. HOW? Easy. Don't let your prime weaknesses through the door. Make a list of the top five foods which make you lose all self-control and send you into a spin of spiralling desire, and prohibit them. Just them. Not everything. Mine are:

✳ **Truffled Camembert**. A provocative rendezvous of oozy cheese and perfumed butter which is quite possibly made by seraphim on a cloud far, far away. If it didn't smell quite so much of cheese I would take it to bed.

✳ **Lindt Orange Intense dark chocolate** – which knows the way to my mouth without even being given directions, let alone a lift.

✳ **Tangy Cheese flavoured Doritos**. These delectable triangles come in a vicious orange packet, and – lo and behold! – they are actually vicious orange themselves, coating your fingertips and lip-corners with a curd of addictive electric dust. Nutritionally objectionable, but my own Achilles snack.

✳ **Jelly Babies**. How couldn't you? Head first!

✳ **Butter**. Like my father and my father's father before me, butter is my downfall, my fridge fantasy. I like it on pretty much anything, as long as it's spread thick, a delicious salty slab of sunny delight. I have even been known to countenance the eating of snails once coated in this glorious substance.

Right, so there's my list. Yours might include – oh, I don't know – crispy bacon, cinnamon buns, flapjacks, Fruit Pastilles, acorn-fed pata negra . . . Whatever your Fat Five, don't allow them a look-in. Sail past them in shops, give them the cold shoulder at parties, bitch about them to your friends. We're not in the business of abnegation. I'm not about to suggest you eat dry toast with a knife and fork while looking daggers at the marmalade pot. But let's be fair here: if you are excising *only* five fattening things, there's still plenty of room for treat eats – just not the ones that will fill your head, your heart and your favourite jeans. I find that a simple swap for a less-loved alternative will cut consumption in half. Unsalted butter has, for me, none of the seductive appeal of the salted stuff; standard Camembert is far less interesting than the truffled variety; I'm safe from the pull of Lindt, as long as I avoid the Orange Intense flavour.

There are certain fiendish foods which just cry out to be eaten. Once you've had a taste, you'll inevitably want more, then more again, as if with each mouthful you weaken even further, until you're reduced to a mess of cookie dough and self-destruction.

Best to note these monsters now, and then treat them with a combination of reticence and respect, as if handling dragons. Your trigger may be a block of Cheddar, a warm loaf, a friendly grab-bag of dairy-milk chocolate. Or fudge. It may be a consoling tub of ice-cream on a bad day. Scones, crisps, biscuits on any day. Yes, we all *know* they're fattening – that's hardly news – but they are also the foods most likely to goad you into hopeless overeating. So, take out the triggers. List them.

Then lose them. Find another less obsessive treat.

56 EXERCISE PORTION PATROL: POLICE THE FOOD ON YOUR PLATE

'If you buy a cookie at a station,' says Dr Tim Lobstein of the International Obesity Task Force, 'it's four inches across! Compare that with the biscuits your granny used to eat. Companies are selling to our eyes rather than to our health needs. And it's only if you read the small print that you can tell what's going on.'

It's true that there has been a portion explosion in the last two decades, leaving the poor punter facing vast hillocks of fodder at every turn, armed only with the vague notion that it is polite to finish up everything on a plate. In their study of why the French remain so much slimmer than Americans, researchers from the University of Pennsylvania came to the remarkable conclusion that it was because the French ate less. The figures – both physically and statistically – back this up. Mean portion size

in Philadelphia was about 25 per cent greater than in Paris.
A supermarket soft drink in the US was 52 per cent larger, a hot-dog 63 per cent larger, a carton of yoghurt 82 per cent larger.
A croissant in Paris weighs one ounce; in Pittsburgh it's two.

Surveys show that one in four Americans eat everything they're served, no matter how enormous it may be. The US is indeed the land of giant pastries, although New York City's Board of Health voted unanimously in March 2008 to require all city chain restaurants to post calorie data on their menus, which may well serve to bring ballooning portions back down to earth. A fascinating study at the University of California's Center for Weight and Health showed that Californians could avoid gaining 2.7 pounds a year if calories were featured on fast-food menu boards state-wide; a voluntary scheme to do just this has recently been introduced in the UK in the hope that knowing how many calories are in your frappuccino or bucket o'wings may well give you pause, or embarrass you into ordering an Evian.

'We face vast hillocks of fodder at every turn, armed only with the vague notion that it's polite to finish everything on a plate.'

It's certainly worth a try. I well remember being overwhelmed by the sheer girth of a muffin I once bought at a coffee shop in Brooklyn – but I braved my way through it under the wayward assumption that it constituted a 'portion' and therefore ought to be finished. This, I later discovered, was a classic behaviour known to psychologists as Unit Bias. 'If food is moderately palatable,' says Paul Rozin, one of the researchers on the Pennsylvania study, 'people tend to consume what is put in front of them, and generally consume more when offered more food.' Interestingly, hamsters do much the same thing.

In another experiment by Professor Brian Wansink at Cornell, subjects were placed in front of a bowl of tomato soup and invited to drink as much as they wanted, unaware that the bowls were being filled covertly from below. A surprising number of people kept right on drinking till the experiment was halted. Was this bottomless greed? Stupidity? Or simple human instinct? Revealingly, Wansink also showed that even *nutritional science professors* ate 50 per cent more soup if it was served in bigger bowls and with bigger spoons.

The issue, then, is that our environment is encouraging idiotic gluttony. Even our glasses have exploded, happily holding three units of Merlot and still leaving room to breathe. In certain restaurants, the wine vessels are virtually impossible to lift without mechanical assistance. Tiffany's top-selling wine glass now holds a profligate 15 fl oz, which is more than enough to send me nose-diving into the salmon starter.

The solution? Read on:

✳ **Take small delicious mouthfuls from small pretty plates.**

✳ **Use your senses.** Think, taste and smell while you eat.

✳ **Leave packaging and food detritus on the table,** in the manner of a Dionysian feast, so you can see at a glance how much you've consumed.

✳ **Use thin glasses** (we tend to pour more into squat ones).

✳ **Buy smaller spoons.**

✳ **Dining out? Sit opposite a mirror.** Eating in? Install one behind your breakfast table. Go subliminal.

✳ You could do worse than remember the *Sex and the City* mantra: **'Order fashionably. Eat sparingly.'**

✳ **Check the small print:** does the lasagne verde sleeve say 'serves four'? Is it trying to tell you something? Do not battle on and eat the lot in one bacchanalian sitting. And do try to remember: the calorie chart on the back may refer to a single serving rather than the whole thing. If it says 'only fifteen calories!' in alluring yellow letters on the front of the packet, look hard until you find the revealing disclosure that this is 'per gram'.

✳ **Decant food into a small and delightful dish,** rather than eating it straight from a box, bag, carton or tub. Put the tub away in a distant cupboard.

✳ **When serving food, leave what great Japanese chefs call 'a margin of emptiness'** at the edge of the plate; this is, says renowned chef Masaru Yamamoto, the 'emptiness of an aesthetic significance, comparable to that in Zen ink painting'.

✳ **Listen up. You don't have to eat everything on your plate.** Really, you don't. The need to clear the plate is what exasperated mothers drum into their pre-schoolers. Unless you are wildly precocious, you are not a pre-schooler. Start taking control of your plate and remember to leave a bit for Mr More.

✳ **Know when to say when, and then say it again.**

✳ **If you fancy seconds, live with that thought for a few minutes,** allowing your stomach to catch up with your mouth. After ten minutes, you're less likely to crave the extra spoonful, no matter how lovin' it looks.

✳ **When you allow yourself a special treat, buy, make and serve individual portions.** So, one toffee, not an entire tablet of fudge. One sorbet in a tub, not a vat of vanilla. A handful of crisps decanted into a single-serve bowl (a ramekin would be ideal), not one of those sacks designed to cater for an extended family at a barbecue.

✳ **Cultivate Tupperware pride:** collect useful receptacles in which to chill or freeze leftovers, rather than plumping for seconds simply to clear a plate. Look upon this as the good, honest, labour-saving, planet-loving, flab-busting endeavour that it is. Label well. You don't want to end up with nameless pots of unidentified matter in the nether world of your fridge.

IDENTIFY WHAT'S IN YOUR TAKEAWAY

Pizza, Indian food and Chinese meals – takeaways in general – are, on the whole, stack-full of calories. Fast food is fat food, so think very carefully before you stroll through the golden arches or pick up the phone. A recent study of 150 takeaways and fast-food outlets for Hampshire County Council found that 'the fat content in a kebab gives you 1,000 calories – equivalent to a wine glass of cooking oil'. Bon ap.

Takeaway	Fat content (grams)	% of GDA*
Doner kebab	139.3	199
Chicken korma	95.4	136
Mixed biryani	100.6	144
Sweet-and-sour pork balls	87	125
Medium pizza and garlic bread	81.5	116
Cornish pasty and chips	74.6	107
Fish and chips	68.5	98
McDonald's Big Mac, large fries†	63	90
KFC, 1 breast, 1 thigh†	44	63
Burger King Whopper†	37	53

*The Guideline Daily Amount (GDA) of fat for women is 70g.
† Data from nutritiondata.com, an authoritative website which gives an accurate nutritional breakdown of thousands of food products. Add it to your Google Favourites and check before you dive into a fast-food feast.

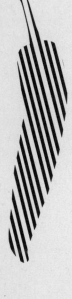

58 READ *FAST FOOD NATION* – YOU MAY NEVER BUY A BURGER AGAIN

'The food revolution of the twentieth century was quite remarkable. How food is grown, cooked, processed, marketed, branded – all this has changed utterly in the past twenty-five years or so. Because we have lived through it, we aren't amazed by it.' So writes Tim Lang, professor of food policy at City University and the man who, years ago, first brought food miles to public attention. To fully appreciate your diet – and by that I mean the stuff you eat, not the stuff you don't eat in order to lose weight – you need an awareness of where it comes from, how it came to be, who benefits from its production and sale. Raising your consciousness by knowing the story behind your food, from farm to fridge to fork, or (possibly) from lab to lunch, will serve to halt your hand as you reach for another Racheroo-Style Potato Wedge.

Today, despite years of re-education, realization and reassessment, plenty of food still comes from the funny farm. If you motor about in the central section of your supermarket, you'll see that little has changed, regardless of the traceability and sustainability arguments which rage at the periphery. I once had a friend whose job it was to 'invent' meat products. We would sit in a bar of an evening, coming up with new versions of mechanically reclaimed protein with which to tempt the market, starting with a snappy name, a packaging proposal and an advertising tag-line. Alas, he was not the man behind Turkey Twizzlers or any such golden goose, but we did spend a good deal of time chortling about the obvious appeal of 'Meat Feet' and 'Chicken Lips', which, as far as I know, never quite got to market. Things may be improving, but we do still have Billy Clown pork luncheon meat (shaped and coloured into a smiley face). In the States, if you're lucky, you can buy 'Potted Meat Food Product' containing *partially defatted cooked pork fatty tissue*. Now, I'm not suggesting this is part of your average daily intake – not knowingly anyway. But plenty of processed food contains suspect ingredients, massive doses of salt and high levels of saturated fat. So think about who really benefits from turning potatoes into waffles and cheese into string. Diverting as they may be, such products are nutritionally corrupt; to digest them at all, our bodies must find the missing minerals, vitamins and enzymes elsewhere – a depletion which, cruelly enough, makes us feel *even hungrier* as our bodies signal for us to replace the nutrients we lack.

Your best defence is to ask the right questions, read the right books, and never again will you be tempted by fake foods. Along with *Fast Food Nation*, try these books for starters: *In Defence of Food: The Myth of Nutrition and the Pleasures of Eating* by Michael Pollan; *Bad Food Britain: How a Nation Ruined Its Appetite* by Joanna Blythman; *Not on the Label: What Really Goes into the Food on your Plate* by Felicity Lawrence. You'll lose weight and gain wisdom.

59 NEVER BE HUNG-OVER – OR STONED

These are the fastest routes to the fry-up and the fridge.

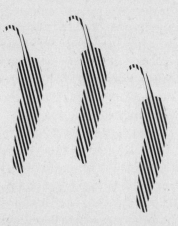
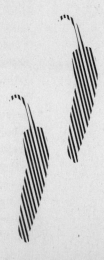

60 DROP THE POP

We all know that Diet Coke is for fat people. But so is fat Coke. Aim for no more fizz, no more 'soda' (such a benign word for such a fiendish thing), and none of that organic elderflower pressé either. Drink water. From a tap. If the tap doesn't turn you on, buy a water filter. Thrill yourself with a slice of lemon, the clink of ice cubes and the thought that it's virtually free. Yes, you have to grow accustomed to the (lack of) taste – but once you do, it's all you'll want.

As you drink, you might like to dwell upon the fact that our taste for diet drinks could be partially responsible for our current obesity problems. Counter-intuitive as it may seem, recent research suggests that consuming zero-calorie sweeteners *increases* the risk of putting on weight. Circumstantial evidence is already convincing: over the past two decades, the number of Americans who regularly eat foods containing sugar-free sweeteners has doubled, while obesity levels have rocketed. But now scientists at Purdue University in Indiana have set about analysing the link. In studies, they found that rats fed yoghurt sweetened with saccharin (a sugar substitute) ate more and grew fatter than those eating yoghurt sweetened with glucose (the real thing).

The researchers posit that sweet foods provide an 'orosensory stimulus' which suggests to the body that a deluge of calories is about to come its way. Like Pavlov's dogs, we've learned that sweet, dense and viscous foods promise lots of lovely calories. When, as with diet drinks, the advertised calories don't materialize, the system becomes confused – and as a result 'people eat more or expend less energy than they otherwise would', says the journal *Behavioural Neuroscience*.

If that's not enough to put you off drinking yourself silly on zero soda, consider too that processed diet foods and no-cal drinks tend to replace fats and sugars with synthetic alternatives and lab-designed nutrients, some of which are known to be toxic. *Toxic!* This is, needless to say, cause for alarm. And the non-diet alternatives? Stacked with sugar. Bad sugar. Fructose – the type of sugar which is found in fruit, but which is also added to fizzy drinks as corn syrup (because it's cheaper than sucrose or glucose) – is more likely than other types of sugar to cause fat to be deposited around your middle. Because fructose is metabolized differently to other sugars, it is also turned at startling speed into body fat.

'Humans, in all our semi-sentient glory, tend to avoid the smallest and largest options when ordering soft drinks, no matter what the volume of that drink may be.'

There's a size issue here too. In an attempt to boost their profit margins, many fast-food restaurants have taken to eliminating smaller drink sizes and adding ever larger ones. A new study suggests that this policy has led to a 15 per cent increase in the consumption of high-calorie drinks – since humans, in all our semi-sentient glory, tend to avoid the smallest and largest options when ordering soft drinks, no matter what the volume of that drink may be. Thus the demand curve shifts ever upward. 'People who purchased a 21-ounce drink when the 32-ounce drink was the largest size available moved up to the 32-ounce drink when a 44-ounce drink was added to the range of drink sizes available,' say the authors. This raises the unedifying prospect of watching a movie accompanied by a 7-Up which requires its own seat. Tsk. So many reasons to ban the can. (Did I mention burping? Or the mark-up on a Pepsi? Your teeth? Do I need to?)

61 ARM YOURSELF AGAINST CALORIE AMBUSH

Your social life is chock-full of reasons to binge. Be prepared by following these fail-safe rules:

At a cocktail party:

✷ **Eat beforehand if you can**, otherwise the canapés will beguile you with their beauty and charm. Pre-eating will also soak up any alcohol coming your way, allowing you to leave the room with decorum and without falling over the doorman.

✷ **If you *have* to eat in situ, go for high-protein canapés.** Try asparagus wrapped in Parma ham, smoked salmon on pumpernickel rye bread, mozzarella and cherry tomatoes, quails' eggs with celery salt, chilli prawns with a zingy lime dressing. Feel free to eat a few low-fat pretzels and anything you find floating in your drink (olive in a martini, mint in a Mojito, celery stick in a bloody Mary, fruit salad in Pimm's).

✷ **Steer clear of cocktail sausages**, even if they are all seductive and sticky with honey and mustard. They are cute but deadly, the hippos of the cocktail scene. Similarly, avoid nachos and their wicked posse of hi-cal dips; also buffalo wings, foie gras, pizza fingers, vol au vents (despite their throwback appeal) and anything made predominantly from cheese.

✷ **Don't station yourself by the swing door to the kitchen in the hope of hoovering up the nibbles.** This is a well-trodden path towards elasticated trousers.

✷ **Don't follow the waiter around the room**, no matter how foxy he may be.

✷ **Don't hover over the canapé platter.** It looks desperate and spreads germs.

✱ **Keep count of what you eat and set yourself a limit** – e.g. five high-protein bites. It's easy to forget how much you've eaten.

✱ **Don't pick up more than you can hold between finger and thumb**. One finger, one thumb.

✱ **Don't let the waiter top up your flute**. Go to the bar. Walk there. Better still, tap dance across the room. Work for that drink.

In a bar. Nuts are high in fat and desperately moreish; the peanut picking which so easily accompanies a gin and tonic is the very enemy of thin, so go without. A few olives are OK at a push. Mini Cheddars? Inadvisable. Tapas, by the way, is still food, even if it comes free with the beer at an authentic Spanish bodega.

At a picnic. This outdoor delight remains one of the few meals still revered in our culture, which is reason enough to indulge. Rushed as we are to eat breakfast on the go, to do lunch in three minutes flat, to get dinner out of the microwave and on to the table, much as we have pushed food to the outer extremes of our lives, the picnic still demands reverie, relaxation. It's a time to linger, to graze.

To keep a lid on this idyllic form of calorie consumption, plan it well. Don't rely too heavily on pork products, that age-old staple of the British picnic rug. Take smoked trout (with horseradish-infused sour cream and a tangle of watercress), turkey breast (a great source of low-fat protein), hard-boiled eggs with a flick of rock salt and imaginative foliage. (Batavia? Radicchio?) Widen your repertoire with, say, toasted couscous, roasted pumpkin, groundnut sprouts, diverting species of radish. Don't just buy it all from Tesco en route to the park.

At a barbecue. It is an irksome fact of life that just as the weather demands that you unveil yourself to all and sundry, so the barbecue season begins in earnest. The traditional meat fest – particularly if undertaken every weekend from mid-June to Labour Day – will leave you looking like a heifer in calf. Instead of burgers, sausages, ribs and wings, go for kebabs with a 60:40 veg-to-meat ratio. If you're the cook, stick some courgette, mushroom, pepper, tomato and onion on there instead of all that meat (for the record, carrots don't work). Go for chargrilled prawns, chilli squid, corn cobs, tuna steaks, a whole fish – bass, bream, trout – baked with dill and lemon juice in a jacket of foil.

At Christmas. Oh, come on! It's Christmas! Live a little. Eat a lot. But do it for one day only. Two, max. The problem with the festive season is that it lasts so very long, each year stretching ever further until soon there won't be a great deal of point in taking down the decorations. Christmas has, as a result, become a gargantuan mother-funster of a feast. Each of us consumes around 6,000 calories on the day itself (eating an average of 3.63 roast potatoes, 2.95 chipolatas and 3.51 desserts, according to a survey by Sainsbury's). Little wonder that the pounds rack up. The way to stop the glut and the gluttony is to Contain Christmas. Let it run amok, but only for a day. Here's how:

✻ **Anticipate festive excess by eating sparingly the week before**; that way, you'll have engineered a deficit, allowing you to splurge with a happy heart.

✻ **Keep in mind that mince pies, Christmas cake, turkey and all its attendant trimmings should be shovelled in on the Big Day itself**, with leftovers making do for Boxing Day. Don't start on the Christmas nosh just because your child has appeared as third donkey in the nativity play. Last year, the nativity play at our school was on 13 November.

✻ **Don't overbuy**, confusing profligacy with hospitality. Go for quality over quantity. Savour, don't hoover.

✻ **Don't eat foods 'invented' for Christmas** – gingerbread in the shape of Christmas trees, Christmas-pudding-flavoured KitKats, turkey-'n'-stuffing-flavour crisps, mulled-wine-flavour cashews, Mr Kipling's Frosty Fancies, chocolate spiked with gold, frankincense and/or myrrh . . .

✻ **Don't keep snack stashes dotted about the house**, fooling yourself that you've got them there in the event of guests. Your mouth is allowed to be empty for part of the festive season, so don't cram your life with additional snacks, whether it's bowls of nuts, bon-bon dishes of Quality Street, dates, walnuts, yoghurt-covered Brazils, chocolate Santas. Hang delightful wooden ornaments on your tree, not cocoa solids.

✱ **Remove all Christmas fare from the house on 27 December**. If you can't make a nutritious soup from it, get rid of it.

At a romantic dinner à deux. You don't need me to suggest you eat moderately. The very act of dining with a potential new boyfriend is a diet on a plate (if only you could have one at every meal). I can confidently predict, therefore, that there'll be no sizzling fajitas, no rib racks, no great tureens of linguine. Basically, you don't want stuff that squirts or dribbles, or anything which requires you to tuck a napkin into your bra. All of which is good from a calorie-cutting perspective. And don't go thinking that ordering tempura is the act of a coquette. It's deep-fat frying, no matter how you dress it up.

At a children's birthday party. I know, I know. There is something exquisitely provocative about the crusts from a Marmite sandwich. I have been known to steal Hula Hoops from the melamine bowls while the kids are occupied with Pass the Parcel. And I have great difficulty handing around the Party Rings without popping a whole one into my mouth and shutting it ever so quickly, like a trap door, leaving me momentarily unable to answer simple questions, such as 'Who ate the last Party Ring?' Hard though it is to accept, stealing food from the mouths of babes is just not on. If you must do it, nick the celery sticks and the carrot batons, which, unlike the Hula Hoops, are generally in plentiful supply.

62 GO ON AN ANTI-HYDROGENATED-FATS DRIVE

I have always been proud of my Italian connection. I like the fact that my great-grandfather was a Florentine milliner called Cesare, a man who would apparently rub raw garlic on a hunk of bread for breakfast and who doused his food in olive oil when the rest of Britain was still only using it to dislodge stubborn ear wax. I like that my grandmother went by the name of Norma Maria Gabriella Annunciata Maranghi, a billowing breath of a name, undulating, lilting, like a swallow flying over the Ponte Vecchio. I love that a small but significant part of me sprang from a country that might not be great shakes at governing itself or keeping tabs on the paperclips, but is so very interested in shoes and handbags and wine and food and art and love. In short, all the good things in life.

Needless to say, an Italian – ancient or modern – wouldn't give house-room to many of the processed foods we salad-dodging Brits consume today in such quantity. There's not a lot of love in artificial cream, no great joy in a dehydrated soup. But you will find other things lurking in there. Like trans fats.

These hydrogenated vegetable oils (HVOs) are unsaturated fatty acids which manufacturers use to give texture ('mouth feel') to food and help preserve it. As Maggie Stanfield points out in her book *Trans Fat*, 'Invented fats of this type are – like natural fats – absorbed into our cell membranes. They fill the space that healthy fats should occupy ... Once the trans fat is in position, it cannot be rejected so the integrity of the cell is compromised. The entire behaviour of the cell alters and this tiny link in the chain of human life, this miniature cuckoo, is empowered to disrupt the whole natural pattern of biological exchange between cells.'

All right, you say, but do they make you *fat*? Stanfield argues that 'it may be that we store trans fats more efficiently and easily. A highly regarded study carried out in North Carolina showed that, even with similar calorie intake, trans fat increases weight gain.'

171

As of July 2008, the city of New York has banned artificial trans fats from its restaurants – and if a conurbation can do it, then you can too. While most UK supermarkets have voluntarily removed HVOs from their own-brand products (with M&S leading the way), they're still there in many branded products, including sweets, stock cubes, frozen meals, takeaways, biscuits, pastries, cereal bars – even vitamin capsules. And they're often not listed in the ingredients. Your best bet is to wean yourself off 'invented foods' altogether. If you fancy going hardcore cold turkey, avoid anything with a long shelf life. You are, after all, not Scott of the Antarctic. Your food doesn't need to withstand a nuclear holocaust. The shops are just up the street – so freshen up and stop opening quite so many hermetically sealed pouches and vacuum-packs. It has been estimated – possibly by a bored student chain-eating Twinkies – that the average person in the West eats over four kilos of food additives every year. To properly redress the balance, go old-school continental. Look for fresh food that's full of life. Rubbing raw garlic on a hunk of bread for breakfast is, of course, optional.

NO GREAT SHAKES:
TIME TO SLASH THE SALT

While you're at it, consider cutting back on salt. According to Eva Longoria's trainer Patrick Murphy, 'Salt is the root of all evil. You can always tell when someone has given it up – their face is thinner, their arms look more toned.' Even if you aren't worried about high blood pressure and heart disease, salt certainly makes you retain fluid, and fluid adds pounds. How to avoid it? Don't add it at the table, go easy on processed foods and discover low-salt soy sauce.

63 READ FOOD LABELS

In a cruel and startling irony, it turns out that plenty of the 'healthy' edibles on our supermarket shelves are no better than the standard full-fat versions. *Which?* magazine, in one of its regular investigative forays, found that Sainsbury's Be Good To Yourself chocolate-chip cookies contained 17 more calories per biscuit than its ordinary variety. A low-fat Oreo apparently has 50 calories; a regular Oreo has 53 calories. This news is thoroughly depressing and likely to drive you straight to the snack cupboard in desperation (come on, I know you've got one).

Most of us already recognize that the modern food-shopping experience is beset by the constant drone of worry . . . *Are we eating enough mackerel? Does mackerel contain mercury? Are there (gulp) any mackerel left in the sea? Wasn't there something about not eating wild? Or was that farmed? And isn't Jemima allergic to fish anyway? But does she eat chicken? And is free-range better than farm-assured? But isn't it a bit unimaginative to serve chicken at a dinner party these days? Shouldn't it be sea trout on a rosti of wild salsify? Is the sun past the yard arm yet? How can it only be quarter to four?*

So here we are, burdened with information and really none the wiser. In fact, as the practice of nutritional labelling on foods has expanded, *so too have our waistlines.* Info-load, far from galvanizing and arming the consumer in the pursuit of health, seems to encourage many of us to tune out. My favourite example of this nannyish state of affairs comes from lawyer Giovanni di Stefano, who recently got a bee in his bonnet about KitKats: 'Do you remember the KitKat?' he said. 'The chocolate bar? Today, when you get the KitKat, it says "open here". Are we that stupid that we can't open a KitKat? If we need someone to tell us "please open KitKat here" – *porca miseria, siamo arrivata allo massimo!* [hell's bells, we've reached the limit!]'

Quite.

In order to assist us in our search for good nutrition, the Food Standards Agency is considering the adoption of 'shock tactics' similar to warnings on cigarette packets, so that dairy snacks, for example, might be emblazoned with graphic images of clogged blood vessels and fatty deposits. These images will have to nestle somewhere alongside the traffic-light system, the list of ingredients, the photograph of the farmer and his dog, the chart showing Percentage of Recommended Daily Allowance, the serving suggestion of the food within, dressed up for best in a fig leaf of coriander . . . By the time you've worked your way through all that, you'll have missed lunch and be hurtling towards supper, questions bouncing around your empty belly.

So, while label-checking is a worthwhile and noble endeavour, don't become a small-print geek, consumed with anxiety and turning food into a trial, not a triumph. If you mull over the nutritional – not to mention the ecological, social and global – significance of every purchase you make, you'll be stuck in the aisle for weeks, paralysed under the fluorescent lights until someone wearing a polyester tunic mops the floor around you. What you really need is a bit of plain common sense, and a couple of trigger words that should make you smell the coffee and run a mile.

✴ **Make sure your supper is mostly food, not mostly numbers**. Would your ancestors recognize your supper? Great. If they'd run a mile, you should too.

✴ **Avoid clearly alien foodstuffs** – 'extruded starch food products', for example. Shun obvious enemies such as high-fructose corn syrup, fractionated palm kernel oil, partially inverted sugar syrup and partially hydrogenated vegetable fat.

✴ **Don't buy anything where the carton weighs more than the product**. As a basic rule, if there is more to throw away than to eat, it's out. If it's dressed like a prom queen, it's out. If you can't tell what it is by looking at it, it's out. If you have to use pliers to get at it, guess what? It's out.

✴ Food, glorious, marvellous **food is pleasure, not poison**. Love it, enjoy it, put in your thumb and pull out a plum.

BEWARE CALORIE CREEP

When the nutritional information on a dozen leading brands a decade ago was compared with the same products today, nine showed an increase in calories, sugar or saturated fat. Researchers found that Kellogg's Rice Krispies contain 36 more calories per 100g than in 1983 – an increase of about 10 per cent. Häagen-Dazs Belgian Chocolate ice-cream contains 16 per cent more calories than in 1994, and 26 per cent more fat. Even products marketed as healthy options are not immune to this 'calorie creep'. According to figures obtained by the *Guardian*, Jordan's Original Crunchy bars have 16 per cent more calories than in 1986, and more fat. Experts say the findings, derived from a comparison of current labels with old ones stored in museum archives, fitted a pattern whereby manufacturers remove salt and some types of fat from food for health reasons, only to compensate with sugar and more fat. 'Reducing salt is an excellent measure, but as a result companies are faced with bland processed food,' explains Tim Lobstein, former director of the Food Commission and now head of the child obesity programme at the International Obesity Task Force. 'The cheap way of flavouring it up is to sugar it. Fat can also help because it helps your tongue notice the flavours – that's why you butter bread,' he says.

The message here is simple enough: despite best intentions, food labelling is not immune to spin. Make sure that you are.

64 WAKE UP IN THE SUPERMARKET

Shopping for food used to be a rather routine and enjoyable exercise. Stroll to corner shop; request pound of tripe; enquire after Ethel's sciatica; pay with enormous five-pound note; return home to mangle the spuds or beat the children. It could happily take all day, what with the chatting and the mangling.

These days – though many of us would dearly like to spend entire Wednesdays sauntering around a farmer's market on the lookout for lavender scones and local lamb shanks – the inevitability is that we'll end up in the supermarket. We'll be lured in by lavishly labelled frozen pizzas and gravy granules, by squeezy mayonnaise and cheap wine.

Yes, a supermarket is convenient and economical and sometimes there's a lady in there giving out free samples of lemon meringue pie. But it's also very often the native habitat of over-processed convenience food and it is designed to suck you in, spin you around and spit you out in the car park having just purchased a three-for-two offer on deep-fill cheesecakes.

Today, 88 per cent of our food comes from the supermarkets, and the very fact that there's so much food, all there, under one vast roof, glinting in its shiny wrappings, simply encourages us to buy (and consume) more. Shopping for food has become a homogenized and strangely hollow experience. On the whole, we're divorced and detached as we purchase our weekly stash – and it is this truncated relationship with food that can be so destructive. Consider for a moment the way we shop at those supermarkets. Like Friesians. Having first stowed our brains in the boot of the car for safe-keeping, we amble about, alighting on items that seem familiar, falling for the sorcery of modern marketing, blinded by gaudy packaging and deafened by the insistent beep of the barcode scanner. Research shows that up to 80 per cent of decisions are made subconsciously as we patrol the aisles. When questioned, some shoppers couldn't remember picking up certain items or didn't know why they had bought them.

Recent studies of the shopping subconscious conclude that many people find shopping a chore, so tend to switch off and act on auto-pilot. People armed with a list of ten things usually bought sixty. 'Of the visual stimuli that assail a shopper,' the study found, 'typically only 1 per cent makes it into the brain's sensory buffer store, and of this, only 5 per cent gets to short-term memory, where it may be matched with previous experience and/or advertising to trigger an emotional response.' It's all a bit Orwellian, isn't it?

Wake up. Right now. Stick to a list. Ignore two-fers and BOGOFs on Jammie Dodgers. If you continue to shop at your favourite supermarket – and there's no doubting that it's easy, reasonable, comforting and relatively painless (unless you're doing it with toddlers in tow) – do try to do it with *awareness*. Or order your groceries online, to avoid temptation. Your bottom line will benefit, in every sense.

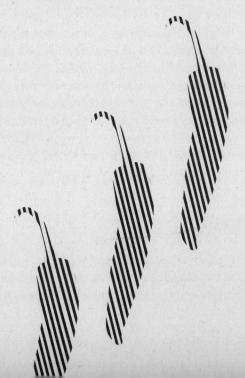

177

65 PUT THE PLATE IN ITS PLACE

If you dream of doughnuts, perhaps you could find something better to feed your fantasies. Look, it's great if your glass is always half full, but if you talk about eating the entire time, discussing lunch at breakfast and dinner at lunch, then it's time to switch your attention to something more uplifting. Here's how to turn yourself off to switch yourself on:

✴ **Meet friends for a walk in the park,** a jog in the gym, a book club, a back rub, not at the tapas bar up the road. Your mouth needn't be full to be having fun.

✴ **Wean yourself off cookery TV.** The food channel is there to inspire, not suck you in for hours and spit you out at bedtime. If you watch a programme on how to make your own pumpkin-and-pine-nut ravioli, dressed with pesto and crispy sage leaves, and then stir yourself from the couch to open a tin of spaghetti hoops, you're missing something vital.

✴ **Fear not an empty fridge.** 'I think that it goes back to the rise of the big American fridge,' says food writer Joanna Blythman. 'It's an aspirational thing.' Indeed it may be, but having great truckles of Cheddar, whole hams and four-tier coffee-walnut gateaux littered about the place is the highway to the wide way. You don't want a completely empty fridge, of course, but something that inhabits the happy middle ground between Spartan and wanton, perhaps containing just enough to see you through a cold snap.

Once you start to think about food in a realistic, rational way, you'll begin to see that you can modify your behaviour around it. You can even playfully push it out of the way. The following may seem a trifle giddy, but they worked for me:

✴ **Discover a fingernail in your favourite brand of muffin (or imagine that you have).** Something similar happened to me with a particularly delicious sandwich of chicken, bacon, mayo – the works – which I had become accustomed to eating every other lunchtime. One day, halfway through this fat-fix, I bit into something rubbery. Bacon? *Euuuuw*, chicken skin? I rolled it about in my mouth. My mouth was perplexed. On examination, it was a sticking plaster. A plaster! In my mouth! Never, never, never again.

✷ **Choose things on the menu you don't fancy much;** it will broaden your palate and your horizons, not your waistline. I once did this with crispy pigs' ears in a posh restaurant in Chiswick. I have done it with snail porridge at Heston Blumenthal's Fat Duck in Bray. I did it with sows' trotters, ducks' hearts and pigs' tails at St John in London, frogs' legs in New Orleans and stir-fried locusts in a back alley in Bangkok, having just had a tattoo of a new moon etched on my shoulder. The point is to view food as an experience – not as comfort, crutch or custom. This investigative, alert relationship with supper is what you're after. Which reminds me of two quotes – one from Wittgenstein (who apparently said, 'I don't mind what I eat, as long as it's always the same thing,' so the great man was clearly a ninny), and the other from Tony Benn, MP. Benn wrote in his diary that he has a thing about triple-cheese pizzas, and has 'eaten two of them every day for years'. Good grief. I want to take the poor man out for a plate of crispy pigs' ears. Rather than settle for the same old, try instead to take your taste-buds on a journey they'll never forget. Besides, if it's locusts for lunch, you're guaranteed not to want seconds.

✷ **Ignore free food.** This includes samples at farmers' markets, chocolate that comes through the post, things on cocktail sticks at conferences, unexpected bonus courses in upmarket restaurants, that half muffin your friend couldn't quite manage ... Fat-traps, the lot of them.

✷ **But for heaven's sake, don't get picky-picky.** Try not to panic if a cream sauce arrives with your fish. A spoonful of sin does not a lard-arse make.

66 BEWARE 'SALARD' AND OTHER HIDDEN FOOD TRAPS

While dodging obvious calorie hazards, it's equally important to avoid apparently 'healthy food' which has been dressed up to the nines: 'salard', for example – defined as a meal which starts out green, good and leafy but soon becomes heavy with cheese, egg, bacon bits, croutons, shards of parmesan, Thousand Island dressing and some leftover chicken wings, all loaded on board in a bid to jazz it up. Similarly, just because the words 'pasta' and 'salad' happen to meet on the side of a takeaway tub, it doesn't mean that this is a salad. It is *cold pasta*. With mayonnaise, flecks of tuna and an afterthought of chopped red pepper. Just as a gym membership card alone will not make you fit, so a meal will not make you thin because it contains broccoli. Use your loaf and stop fibbing.

But before you head off to the salad bar like a beatified martyr, you may also like to consider this: according to a series of studies at Cornell University, 'the "health halos" of healthy restaurants often prompt consumers to treat themselves to higher-calorie side dishes, drinks or desserts than when they eat at fast-food restaurants that make no such health claims.' The findings, published in the *Journal of Consumer Research*, reveal that people also tend to underestimate by up to 35 per cent just how many calories so-called healthy foods contain. The answer is to go easy. Don't cram. And don't sneak in a Snickers as a prize because you've had a falafel wrap which contained grated carrot. I know you. I'm watching.

67 DRINK LESS ALCOHOL

It's eight p.m. End of a long day. Traffic jam. Tax man. PMT. VAT. Irritating acronyms. Irritating husbands. That bloke in front of you at the post office who was turning his pennies into pounds. *Sheez*, no wonder you're tired, frazzled. The sofa is all set to give you a hug. But first? First, you'll open a bottle of wine.

Course you will. We all do it. That nightly bottle of Shiraz or Chardonnay has become the comfort of a generation. Most women I know spend regular evenings in with Ernst and Julio Gallo, occasionally flirting with an audacious Wolf Blass or a muscular Tim Adams. Our grandparents, you may remember, drank wine, if at all, as a treat. They may have had sherry in the sideboard, a G&T in the garden and sweet liqueurs, all sticky label and curdy cork, available for the resuscitation of elderly visitors. Sure, they had the pub for a pint, a port and a pickled egg. But they didn't have wine by routine, night in, night out, with barely a night off.

Plenty of us do today, though. While forty-somethings indulge at home, many twenty-somethings are out on the razz, bingeing on booze till they hurl. Medical implications aside, this is an epic disaster for weight management. So now is the time to bid the bottle adieu, not for ever, but perhaps just Monday to Thursday. Instead of having a nightly blow-out on plonk, come home to a simple omelette, a knot of deep-green watercress and a single great glass of good wine. Something to savour. You'll gain so much – and here's what you'll lose: the morning headaches, the groggy half-sleep during breakfast, the dehydrated mouth on the Tube, the half-stone which has settled on your middle like a lazy pet dog . . .

It's well worth doing. Official figures have recently revealed that millions of affluent, middle-class women are drinking far more alcohol than they think. It's all slipping down a treat, without unduly upsetting the conscience (or the neighbours). According to the British Dietetic Association, this behavioural shift has given British women a whole new shape – an unexpectedly fitting 'wine-glass figure'. The increase in alcohol consumption among females has apparently caused us to accumulate weight less around bums and tums (be grateful for small mercies), but more around the middle, similar to the traditional beer belly on men. You don't need to be told that this is not a good look. Nor is it a healthy one. Mark Bellis, director of the North West Public Health Observatory, which has been monitoring this low-key binge-drinking among Britain's middle classes, says, 'Across England around one in five adults is drinking enough to put their health at significant risk and one in twenty enough to make disease related to alcohol consumption practically inevitable.' Hmm. While the health implications should give us all pause as we reach again for the corkscrew, the weight factor is perhaps more immediate and compelling, and we'd do well to sober up and face the facts of our nightly fix before we're all built more like beer barrels than wine glasses.

All drinks were not created equal, so it's time to crack down on the fatteners and go slim-line. Luckily, some spirits – tequila, gin and vodka – contain no carbs. That is not to say that they contain no calories, but it does mean that they are preferable to downing great vats of vino, which can really stack up if you're not concentrating. Clearly, the very point of alcohol is that you soon stop concentrating, allowing you to wander the streets late at night falling into hedges and singing 'Danny Boy' to the lamp-posts. In weight-loss terms, this is hopeless. Drink not only inhibits sleep, it stimulates appetite (which is surely the only reason the doner kebab persists in our culture). Nutritionists recognize that the body processes alcohol before it gets to work on fats, proteins and carbohydrates – which means drinking slows down the burning of fat. Worse still, it reduces inhibitions, allowing you to do crazy things, such as finding out how many M&Ms you can fit into your mouth in one go. Hilarious, yes, but not if you're aiming to fit into that bikini any time soon.

Bear in mind, too, that a glass of wine used to be one unit; now – thanks to those generous glass sizes – it's two. If you insist on having a drink, a few pointers:

✳ **Stop drinking dry white.** Start drinking vodka (but not in the same quantities).

✳ **Keep adding ice cubes.**

✳ **Sip. And spritz.**

✳ **Choose small glasses;** fill halfway, in the manner of a top-flight sommelier.

✳ **Keep the opened wine bottle in the fridge or in a seldom-seen cupboard,** so that, should you wish to refill your glass, you need to set out on an expedition.

✳ **If you *have* to snack while drinking, avoid salty stuff:** it makes you thirsty, so you drink more (which is why the pub trade loves a peanut).

✳ **Educate your mouth:** train your palate to appreciate fine wine and reject appalling old plonk. Buy one great bottle and savour it.

✳ **Make every second drink water.**

✳ **Watch your mixers.** Club soda, lemon and lime juice are the best bet; a cheeky orange juice will double the calorie count of a vodka shot.

✳ If, like me, you're in the habit of pouring yourself a very generous glass of Pinot Gris as soon as your children are snoring gently in their cots, you will get through a serious number of units over the course of an average week. **Introduce TT nights –** say, Monday to Thursday – when you lay off the booze completely. You could halve your weekly alcohol intake this way; you'll also slash your liquid calorie consumption, wake up with a spring in your step, cut back on your shopping bill, and – if you're anything like my friend Dan – start that novel you've always been meaning to write. Personally, I have taken up the piano and now play *Für Elise* on such a loop each evening that I am annoying the neighbours.

A BIG NIGHT OUT?

Alcohol has around seven calories per gram, making it twice as fattening as protein or carbs, and almost as calorific as fat. Interestingly, a martini has about the same number of calories as a slice of cheese pizza. Calories in drink are sad and 'empty', being of no earthly value to your poor beleaguered body, apart from making it feel momentarily irresistible. The truth will out by daybreak, trust me.

Drink	Carbs	Calories
Beer (12 fl oz)	13	140–160
Red wine (5 fl oz)	4	122
White wine (5 fl oz)	5	118
Champange (4 fl oz)	1.2	78
Whisky (1 fl oz)	0	64
Tequila (1 fl oz)	0	65
Vodka (1 fl oz)	0	65
Gin (1 fl oz)	0	65
Lemon juice (1 tbsp)	1.3	4
Lime juice (1 tbsp)	1.4	4
Orange juice (0.5 cup)	13.4	56
Tomato juice (0.5 cup)	5.1	21

HOW TO MIX THE
PERFECT DRY MARTINI

If I am going to indulge, I want to make it something memorable. Something glamorous. Something like a martini. The marriage of gin and vermouth is not only classically chic, it is an alchemy of flavours which is entirely magical. How could a pizza compete? Here's how to do it right:

*Ignore Bond's advice. A dry martini *must* be gin-based; vodka is inert in the presence of vermouth, which makes it nothing but a mouthful of boredom.

*Ensure that everything is sub-zero cold. Freeze first.

*Pour a hint of vermouth into an ice-filled shaker. I said a hint. Not a slosh. Connoisseurs call for a fifteenth of the quantity of gin you intend to use. I prefer a seventh.

*Stir. Don't shake. 007 really was a double-oh-ditz when it came to martini-making (shaking adds way too much water and obscures the point of this drink).

*Discard the vermouth; enough of what you need is clinging to the ice. Decadent isn't the word.

*Add your chosen gin, and a drop of Angostura Bitters if you're that way inclined. Stir again and serve.

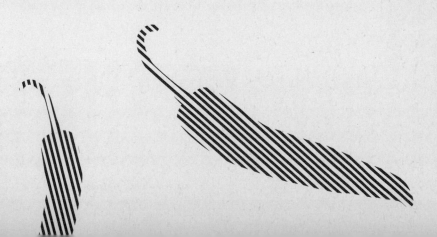

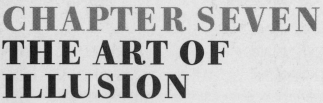

CHAPTER SEVEN
THE ART OF ILLUSION
Diversion, Distraction and Deception

So here we are at the heart of the beast. You've already made brilliant progress by eating well, engaging more, judging less. Excellent. Now it's time to fake it. These canny moves, gleaned from my years in the fashion industry, will unveil the slim new you in seconds, without any need to deny yourself a decent lunch. You'll discover ways to shave off an inch here, a bulge there; ways to run interference so that your assets get all the attention and your liabilities sneak under the radar; ways to fib and flatter so you'll never need to diet again. Once you've tried them, you'll love them for life. Here, then, are the tricks of the trade.

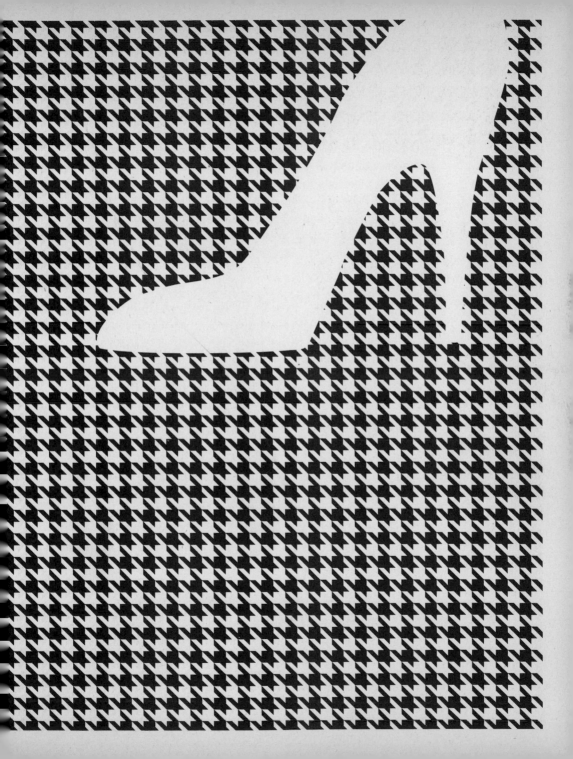

68 WEAR HEELS

'Good heavens!' said my father not long ago, shocked enough
to keep his espresso hovering just below his lower lip. 'That is
the first time I have ever seen you wearing flat shoes!'

He wasn't being strictly accurate, of course, unless I sprang
from the womb wearing a nice pair of Manolo Blahnik sling-backs
(anything is possible, I grant you, given my lifelong predilection
for heels). I do believe I wore flats to come third in the hundred-
metre dash in 1976, and again to climb Mount Snowdon by
mistake in 1992 (we took the wrong path in the mist and arrived
at the summit entirely by accident. I had thought I was popping
out to buy a Fruit & Nut).

But, in principle, my dad was right. I am indeed rarely out of
heels. There are people I have known for years who have no idea
how tall I am. I have worn platforms on the beach at St Tropez. I
have driven all the way to Cumbria in a finicky pair of complicated
stilettos (my, how the locals chortled when I arrived at the pub).
My feet are so used to living at a 45-degree angle that I feel giddy
on the flat, like Ellen MacArthur just off the yacht.

In this respect, I am much like Victoria Beckham, who
apparently 'can't concentrate in flats' (though my all-time
favourite quote on the subject comes from Mariah Carey, who
says, 'I can't wear flat shoes. My feet repel them'). From our lofty
perspective, there is no earthly point in a flattie. 'Why,' I asked
my lanky friend Veronica, 'would you want to slap through life,
your feet flapping about like Olive Oyl's, making a noise like rump
steak on lino, when you could teeter and totter about like a foal?'

'Because,' retorted Veronica, 'women in stupid bloody heels look
vaguely incapacitated at all times, as if mid-swoon and expecting
a man to leap to their defence.'

She's not keen on being manhandled, Veronica. But she has
a point. The wearing of high heels is perhaps the last bastion of
unreconstructed anti-feminism left in our wardrobes, and one
which many of us embrace so willingly. Yet we all know that high
heels hurt. They send our pudenda forward (if we're walking like

a catwalk queen) or our asses out (if we're not). They compromise our spines and trash our very soles. They are hazardous to ankles. They ruin hardwood floors. Proper high heels, incidentally, are also fiercely expensive. But still we love them so.

We love them because they are a short-cut to sizzle. Superlative shoes can add sex to any outfit, regardless (and this is the crux) of the body which sits on top of them. They also trick the eye into elongating the leg, making you look instantly thinner. In my fattest, darkest moments, a pair of Sergio Rossi tomato-red sling-backs has dragged me from the depths. When pregnant and built like a prize-winning pumpkin, Manolos got me through. As most canny women know, vertiginous heels are the fairy-dust that turns jeans into dynamite, tailored trousers into rock 'n' roll cool, pumpkins into princesses.

For Nicole Kidman, a woman of five foot ten forced into humbling flats for the duration of her marriage to Tom Cruise (five foot seven), heels were a liberation. 'Now I can wear heels,' she sighed as their divorce came through, and what she meant was 'Now I am free.' For others, they mean 'Now I am rich.' Look at Elizabeth Hurley, Victoria Beckham, Paris Hilton, their feet routinely housed in non-shoes made from angel breath and unicorn hair, proclaiming to onlookers that they never have far to walk. Interestingly, Victoria Beckham wears those strappy shoes way beyond the red carpet; she wears them to attend football matches, to traipse through airports, to trawl the world's prime retail acreage. She wears her glass slippers long after the ball; she wears sandals in a snowstorm. Today, bizarrely, this is the mark of the prodigiously rich.

A shoe, then, is no mere afterthought: whether you are a Posh or a prole, it is the basis of your day, plotting the curve of your spine and the wiggle in your walk (I need hardly remind you that Marilyn Monroe had her Salvatore Ferragamo shoes made with one heel lower than the other, to lend that reckless roll to her gait). There is, when you stop to stare, so much cargo in those meagre scraps of leather, so many messages transmitted by tongue and sole. If you get your shoes on side, right now, then you're partway to thin-dressing and you haven't even pulled up a zipper yet. Next time you sling on your shoes as you rush for the door, choose with care. Choose a heel. Lose a pound.

THE DON'TS AND DOS OF SHOES

Footwear is no afterthought. It is the very basis of smart dressing, and your platform for change. Some shoes will cleverly, graciously, whittle away the weight, while others will only add to your excess baggage. It pays to know precisely what a shoe can do for you, so accompany me now on a journey through the highs and lows of heels:

✳ **Sling-back**. The most seductive of shoes, chiefly because the strap is ever perilously close to collapse, leaving you – *swoon* – naked from the ankle down. They're a bit *déshabillé*, sling-backs, and thus hopelessly sexy. They also have an illusion going on, leading the eye all the way from hem to toe without any troublesome obstacle, unlike the . . .

✳ **Ankle-strap** – which, by some freak of design, will effectively chop your legs off before they've finished. Needless to say, this is absolutely not advisable if you're after a long, lean look. Wear only when at the very pitch of fashion (for about ten minutes every third year). Otherwise steer clear and go instead for the . . .

✳ **Gladiator**. Yup, the ancient shoe that wouldn't die. There is something very appealing about a whip of leather pirouetting up a shin. Reminiscent of corsetry, with a mild fetish overtone, gladiators – flat or high – manage to make a calf look contained, and thus slimmer, avoiding the ankle-strap trap by encouraging the eye ever up rather than stopping it dead in its tracks. What's more, gladiators which chase up a leg manage to disguise a multitude of sins (varicose veins, stubble, unsightly blotchiness). All good, I hear you cry, throwing down this book to get your mitts on a pair. Well, yee-es. But a word of warning: do beware the sun. Lattice-striped shins will make you look like a gala pie, which is almost as bad as a . . .

✦ **Round toe**. Why? Because a stumpy toe can easily give the impression that you are plodding about on trotters, stealing an inch or more of length from your frame. Add an ankle-strap and you have the world's most fattening shoe. Apart from the . . .

✦ **Ballet pump**. Worn with the wrong clothes, the ballet pump nicks the biscuit. I have one pair of red pumps that my husband calls my 'fat shoes', which somehow takes the shine off wearing them. With a full skirt they make me look several orders wider. They do, however, look marvellous with Capri pants, a marriage made in style heaven, as dear Audrey Hepburn demonstrated so prettily. My most treasured ballet pumps are in silver, which only adds to their allure. (I'm debating the purchase of the gold, which might just be a gesture too far, like having gilt taps in your en suite.) Anyhow, the rule is to wear ballet pumps with slim-line trousers – cigarette pants, Capris, skinny jeans, that kind of thing. Wear them with a dirndl skirt and it's curtains. What you really need with a swishy skirt is a . . .

✦ **Kitten heel**. These darling shoes manage the tightrope walk of making your feet look adorable and petite, while allowing them to perch on a reasonably low, stable heel. This is a plus for any woman who actually has to walk between engagements. They are, however, one of those shoes that tiptoes into fashion from time to time, rather than being a constant companion. If kitten heels don't seem on trend this season, settle instead for a . . .

✦ **Pointed toe**. Oh, do I really need to tell you how vampish and gorgeous they are? Not ideal if they are out of fashion, as is occasionally the case (you'll look like a madam), but they truly triumph if they are on trend. Go for a toe that could puncture tyres and a heel that promises death to all invertebrates foolish enough to cross your path. Wearing them regularly may, of course, make your feet look like they've been beaten with a rolling pin. But what the heck! Winkle-pickers care little for comfort. They rock, they roll, but they certainly don't buy you flowers and ask after your health. They do, however, manage the dual feat of elongating the leg *and* slimming the ankle, while giving passing

191

blokes the impression that you will not take it lying down.
A similar effect may be obtained from a . . .

✳ **Peep toe**. Though to my mind, this other leftover from a bygone age is a mere also-ran which ought to be stamped out, chiefly (though inexplicably) because it gives the strong suggestion that you have just stubbed your toe. The peep toe is also faintly daft, a design detail too far. Why does your middle toe need a sun roof? If your feet are hot, wear . . .

✳ **Strappy sandals**. Yes, they are the preserve of the super rich, worn by the limo classes and quite a number of bawdy strumpets out on the lash on a Friday night. But still. Who wouldn't? Says Paola Jacobbi, author of *I Want Those Shoes*, 'Look at sandals – they are the bikini of footwear . . . you can be fully dressed but in some way you are naked; you can wear strappy sandals and your whole look is subverted. That's why women will wear them even when it is cold or they have to walk far.' The rule here is to wear them only if you own decent feet. No corns, bunions, verrucas, calluses, or any other objectionable. If your feet leak out between the straps, please return them to the tissue-interior of the box and opt instead for an . . .

✳ **Ankle boot**. These little pixies have been hogging the limelight lately, and with good reason. Half-shoe, half-boot, the versatile hybrid waltzes through the seasons like there's no tomorrow. My own favourite is the 'shoot', the upshot of a midnight encounter between a shoe and a boot, resulting in a crossbreed which looks a treat under trousers and still manages to walk the walk with tights and a skirt. On the whole, however, anyone with generous calves really ought to see sense and recognize that an ankle boot will make them look like Nellie the Dancing Elephant. Far better to go with a . . .

✳ **Knee-high boot**. There is, after all, something dashing about a really great boot. Flat riders, bikers, cowboys . . . piratical, slim-line, zipped, elasticated . . . it matters little what you choose. These heroes will cradle your legs and pilfer a couple of centimetres from their circumference. If you can't find a boot to fit, try a specialist website such as duoboots.com, which has thirty-three styles in twenty-one different calf and foot sizes. If it's height you're looking for, though, you'll be wanting a . . .

Platform. Hopeless in a hurry, but a perennial favourite. I have loved them for decades. My very first platform shoes were bought for me during that long, hot summer of '76. They were easily as high as they were long, decorated in floral-sprigged cotton, and impossibly dangerous for a nine-year-old child to negotiate. It was like having a couple of pocket dictionaries attached to my junior-school feet – and even today, I am amazed that my mother (who made me wear two pairs of pants on cold days) allowed me to have them at all. Still, a love story started then, and to this day I'm a fan. Platforms, you see, are a great way to add length without the demanding tightrope walk of a proper stillie. Bear in mind that they are, by nature, blocky and can easily make you seem bottom heavy, strapped to the ground like Neil Armstrong on the moon. Avoid enormous stack heels of the kind which could unwittingly flatten small children. If in doubt, try a . . .

Wedge. Again, you'll acquire an illusion of stature with less wobble than a skinny heel, thanks to a broader, safer centre of gravity. Perfect for the navigation of grass, gratings, the lawns of country-house hotels during wedding receptions, cobblestones outside the pub, cattle grids during short walks in rural areas, and significantly more interesting than the . . .

Court. There are several ways to go with this one. Play safe (navy, mid-height, block heel) and you will look like a local-government admin assistant. Not that there's anything wrong in that as such. But if you are on the hunt for a little *ooh*, a little *aah* and a whole lot of thin, you'd do better to raise up and slim down that heel. Always avoid fat heels. Fat heels = fat feet. Black and navy shoes are, incidentally, about as interesting as . . . as . . . yawn, sorry, too bored to even come up with a simile.

Let's move on.

69 FIND YOUR WAIST AND CHERISH IT

And so to the tricky issue of high-rise versus low-rise waists. It's one of those perennial issues of fashion, and you'll already know which camp you favour. But are you doing yourself any favours? Should you reconsider?

First, a word in favour of high-rise trousers. Erin O'Connor looks absolutely amazing in them. She looks like a sapling, a human exclamation mark. If anything, they make her look taller and more elegant than she really is. And this woman is *tall*. She makes Kate Moss look like an occasional table. On such a slender ribbon of a thing, the effect of a high waist can be dynamite. I once shared a Parisian taxi with Erin, zipping between fashion shows, and this girl is collapsible, like a garden chair. She seems to fold telescopically in the middle, allowing her to occupy cramped spaces, such as the back seat of a Peugeot 206.

For those of us burdened with a tummy, the high-waist trouser is, by stark contrast, nothing but a blight. If, like me, you are more curve than taper, they will do you no favours at all, apart from, perhaps, keeping that roly-poly tummy of yours warm in a draught. Should you insist on tapping this trend, however, take some tips. Number one: always wear with heels. Gorgeous high heels which require you to sit down often (practise doing the Erin foldaway-chair routine). Two: make sure your high-risers are made from slim-line fabric, not the kind of thickening tweed that will make you look more trunk than sapling. And three: *breathe in* if someone threatens to take your photograph.

Your alternative is to stick with the groovy rock 'n' roll lounge look of the low-rise trouser, which can do much to elongate a dumpy, stumpy sort of figure. Mind you, low-slung has its issues too. Butt cleavage, for one (Hello moon!), which is frankly rude in mixed company, or the ludicrous sight of a thong peering out above a waistband as if looking for predators. Sarah Jessica Parker, herself an arbiter of style and doll-sized to boot, told *Vogue* some time ago that she doesn't consider low-rise pants to be age-appropriate for a woman such as herself. It's up to you to make that choice, but do bear in mind that alighting on your waist and making a point of it is one sure-fire way to look immediately slimmer.

BABY, BABY, WHERE DID YOUR WAIST GO?

In 1951 – according to the last government-sponsored sizing survey – the average woman had a 27.5-inch waist. By 2004, according to Size UK findings, it had expanded to 34 inches – that's an inch a decade and counting. This points up the intriguing paradox that while we are desperate to keep up with our ever-shrinking celebrities, the average woman is getting wider. (You'll know this if the old romantic in you has ever tried to cram itself into your grandmother's wedding dress.) 'Women resemble men much more so than they did in the fifties,' confirms Jeni Bougourd, senior research fellow at the London College of Fashion. 'While we are bigger overall, the waist has grown more, in proportion. Modern women are very much straighter now.'

Quite why this is happening may seem obvious. We eat too much. But it's not just about quantity. Says Emma Stiles, nutritional scientist at the University of Westminster, 'The waist–hip ratio has changed over the last hundred years because of a change in the macronutrients in our diet. Our intake of carbohydrates and sugars has grown rapidly, which increases insulin production. This in turn aids fat-cell deposits on the torso rather than anywhere else on the body.' It turns out that while our celebrity icons threaten to slip between the cracks in the pavement, the rest of us are busy becoming bollards. If we resemble anyone these days, it's not Posh Spice. It's Elton John.

How, then, to deal with this thickening? Eat less, sure. But you can cheat, too:

✳ A wide belt will keep your tummy under control and do the job of a corset if you find the latter a bit Miss Whiplash.

✴ A cummerbund is no sin with a superior smoking jacket.

✴ A wrap dress, a ballet cardigan, a wide sash tied in a bow like a Christmas Eve surprise? All great ways to make your waist work and leave your bottom out of proceedings.

✴ Pick out designers who really know how to throw a curve at a woman's body. Roland Mouret, for instance. His long-loved Galaxy dresses, and many of his more recent creations, are underpinned by a canvas, boned 'waist restrainer', with a metal-toothed zip up the back for support. Victoria Beckham has pulled a similar stunt with her Dress Collection.

✴ Another way to fake it is by working not on your overall shape, but on your proportions. 'Modern women are looking at the waistlines in the magazines and thinking, "Oh, crikey, how am I going to wear this?"' a fashion buyer once told me. 'To create that tiny waist today, given our new proportions, you have to cheat, by giving volume to the skirt and cropping the jacket higher.' Got that?

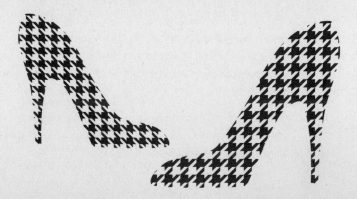

70 MASTER OPTICAL ILLUSION

There's so much to remember. I suggest you photocopy this bit and stow it in your handbag:

✱ A V-neck will lend your body a subtle vertical line. This is good.

✱ A turtle-neck, though, will make you look like a turtle. This is bad.

✱ Flared legs will balance fuller tops. That's trouser legs, not *your* legs.

✱ A shrunken jacket makes everything look smaller – but not if your bottom is vast.

✱ If your bottom *is* vast, a drop-waist skirt will minimize it.

✱ Similarly, an A-line will endeavour to make a big bottom smaller, chiefly by leaving it well alone. Do be aware that an A-line can easily turn into a tent. Try before you buy.

✱ Wear a long silky print scarf to elongate a figure. Not a fat cravat. A thin Isadora Duncan, please (avoid vintage-car rallies).

✱ Extreme heels will slim an ankle. Doh.

✱ A long necklace, à la Coco Chanel's pearls, will lengthen the torso and enhance a cleavage.

✱ A wide belt will define your waist and give it shape. Not too tight, mind. It shouldn't look uncomfortable, like a twist in a sausage.

✱ A high-waist skirt in a supportive fabric will streamline the tummy (as Nigella Lawson will confirm). The trick here is to wear your heels and your collar high to create a sinuous, endless silhouette.

✱ Chokers will slim down a medium-sized neck. NB, chokers will choke a very thick neck. Let your mirror (and your ability to breathe) be your guide.

✳ If you have heavy thighs, an empire line – belted or ribboned – can accentuate your narrowest part. Do this. Do it now. Beware, however, the unfathomable pull of the baby-doll dress. An empire needs to be sleek and assured. It does not need to suck its thumb and ask for a lollipop.

✳ A front crease in tailored trousers will elongate the leg; back pockets will slim a big bottom.

✳ Peg-front trousers are suspect (at least if you want to look thinner). The additional fabric adds bulk and makes you look like the keyboardist from A-ha. Go for flat fronts, which keep everything nicely tucked in.

✳ Trousers with a cuff or turn-up tend to shorten the leg.

✳ Black shoes with black opaques will make your legs go on for miles. Ditto tanned legs and nude shoes.

✳ If you are blocky, break up the broads with a contrasting mid panel; a long scarf, or a black jacket over a light-coloured tee, will perform a similar trick.

✳ Floaty layers are usually kind to bulges. Don't go too frou-frou though, or you'll look like a Portuguese man-of-war.

✳ Velvet and corduroy tend to thicken a body by reflecting light. You get the same effect from carpets.

✳ Similarly, shiny fabrics make you look bigger, which is why cyclists should wear them and women in search of elegance should not.

✳ A two-piece, two-colour outfit – your skirt navy and your jacket beige, say – is gopping. It will skew your proportions and incite a fight between your upper and lower halves. When planning an ensemble, go for something that elongates your figure, taking the eye on an exquisite journey from halo to toenail, *not* something that chops you up like a magician's assistant.

✱ A twin set, however, is an absolute *gift* of optical illusion: the shell bit clings to your frame (great), while the cardigan offers camouflage, comfort and shelter in a stiff wind. It also distracts the eye from an ample belly. Brilliant. Be patient; they'll be back.

✱ If you have pockets, keep them empty. Seriously. What earthly point is there in buying expensive handbags (which I urge you to do – it's just such *fun*), if you insist on keeping your mobile, your lipstick, your shopping lists and a few Prussian pfennigs in your pocket? A full pocket is like a full nappy. Objectionable in the extreme.

✱ I like this tip from Sir Paul Smith, a man who knows a very great deal about successful dressing: 'If you have a big bust, stick to single-breasted blazers to avoid adding volume. Longer-line jackets flatten rounder hips. High heels, rolled-up sleeves and pretty jewellery will stop this look becoming too masculine.'

✱ And this, from Betty Jackson on dressing curves: 'To find your ideal summer dress, look in a mirror at the area between the collarbones. Anything that drapes, knots, tucks, crosses or folds along that vertical body line (be it high or low neck) will disguise problems brilliantly – particularly if it's flattened down by stitching. These design details will shave off inches while allowing ease of movement and look really elegant.'

'An empire needs to be sleek and assured.
It does not need to suck its thumb and ask
for a lollipop.'

THE UPS AND DOWNS OF STRIPES

A word about vertical stripes. I know, dull, dull, dull, but they work ... Or do they? In a spot of sensational myth-busting, psychologists at York University have found that up-down stripes are more fattening than hoops. In the study, volunteers looked at two hundred pairs of images of women in several sorts of stripe. Horizontal stripes were judged to be significantly more slimming. (To make the women in the pictures appear to be the same size, the ones wearing the horizontal stripes had to be 6 per cent wider.)

Dr Peter Thompson, who led the research, is mystified as to how we could have got it so wrong, pointing out that scientists have been aware of the unflattering properties of vertical stripes ever since German physiologist Hermann von Helmholtz created his 'squares illusion' in the 1860s. Von Helmholtz drew two identically sized squares and put vertical stripes on one and horizontal stripes on the other; the square with the horizontal stripes appeared taller and thinner than the other square, prompting Helmholtz to note that 'ladies' frocks with cross stripes on them make the figure look taller'.

In truth, stripes of any persuasion can be challenging. Though chic, they distort in a very obvious way when navigating a bulge, which is a bit like drawing an arrow on your belly and asking people to throw it commiserative glances. If you're keen on stripes, go matelot (the brilliant sailor-top classic which has Deauville sewn into its seams) or widen the stripes for a punky punch. Do try not to wear vertical candy-stripes, though, particularly in Brighton, where people might pay to sit on you.

71 WEAR INTERESTING AND DIVERTING ACCESSORIES

✱ If at all possible, buy diamonds.

✱ Otherwise, go for thumping great accessories – like those vast handbags and sunglasses worn by Paris Hilton, Lindsay Lohan and Victoria Beckham. Not only will you look thinner, but you'll burn calories as you lug them all around. Genius. So good, in fact, that *Marie Claire* was prompted to call the idea 'one of its top diet tips for summer'. You can achieve the same dwarfing effect with huge DJ-style headphones, roller skates or a very big boyfriend.

✱ Never embellish a problem area, hoping to disguise it. You may as well stick on a false moustache and kiss your ass goodbye. If you have an ample chest, avoid breast pockets and double-breasted jackets. If you're wider than you'd like, steer clear of side pockets, peplums and panniers, unless you are auditioning for a role in *School for Scandal*.

✱ Bows, frills and ruffles are not interesting and diverting accessories. They are haberdashery and ought to be confined to the dressing-up box, or at the very least conferred upon someone who might find them useful, such as Keira Knightley. My Great-Aunt Betty, a substantial woman in every sense, habitually wore flamenco frills, most often in the colours of international flags. She forever looked like a galleon in full sail, or a pair of Austrian blinds cruising up the hallway en route to the nearest box of Milk Tray. If fashion dictates ruffles, find your inner anarchist and tell fashion to eff off. Quote Leonardo da Vinci to shore up the argument: 'Simplicity,' he said, 'is the ultimate sophistication.' (See diamonds, above.)

✱ Stall the audience at ground level. Blissfully, most design houses have got into the swing of producing shoes mad enough to be certifiable, which makes them both conversation pieces and a terrific diversionary tactic. Shoes are becoming more and more delirious, as if afflicted by a cumulative condition that will one day send them over the edge in a flailing hail of sequins and lizard skin. Choose from the feathered, mirrored and patent; go for colour, texture, tantalizing heel shapes. If Prada's hand-sculpted shoes don't train the eye off a bountiful bottom, I don't know what will.

'Shoes are becoming more and more delirious, as if afflicted by a cumulative condition that will one day send them over the edge in a flailing hail of sequins and lizard skin.'

72 KNOW THE ENDURING STRENGTH OF BLACK

Now I recognize it's not fun with a capital F, but if you really want to slim your booty, the very best way to do it is to discover the enduring power of black and navy (and, to a lesser degree, neutrals). Dull? Possibly. Dense? Fair point. Effective? Hell, yes.

Despite criticism that wearing black tends to weigh down a figure and disguise curves – breasts, for example, which can be a delightful addition to a silhouette – the bare fact is that black is a thinning agent. If you transport yourself for a moment back to the physics lab of your past, you'll remember that white reflects light and makes things look larger (think of a room); black absorbs light and makes things look smaller. Yippie-ka-yay! Johnny Cash was really on to something, as Dr Peter Thompson, psychologist at the University of York, confirmed in a recent experiment: 'Wearing black is a good thing,' he concluded. 'That one works. We looked at a black circle on a white background and a white circle on a black background. The black circle looked smaller than the white one.'

It is this reliable optical illusion which perhaps explains why a recent survey found that 41 per cent of our wardrobes are made up of black clothes. We each of us, on average, own five black coats, two LBDs and twelve pairs of black shoes. No wonder our partners rarely notice if we've been out on a shopping splurge; marvellously, it really *does* all look the same to the untrained eye.

I checked my own wardrobe against these figures – breaking down my formidable closet into colour-coded zones, a bit like the car park at Ikea. I was amused to discover that 70 per cent of my wardrobe is resolutely black, and a further sizeable chunk is navy-blue, which is little more than a coy excuse for black. On the shoe front, from trainers to towering stilettos, I own thirty-six pairs of black shoes. I found, to my astonishment, that I actually possess two identical pairs of black ballet pumps, which I have been wearing for three years thinking they were one and the same pair. And as for Little Black Dresses? My evening wardrobe has relied for so long on the forgiveness and chivalry of black that I can lay claim to only three posh dresses that contain any colour at all – and one of those was bought for a fancy-dress party when I (unfathomably) decided to go as Elizabeth Taylor in *Who's Afraid of Virginia Woolf?* The rest is black to the bones.

Since this tends to look funereal, as if all your clothes have gathered for a wake, it is worth spiking it up with jolts of colour, flashes of flesh and the occasional print, if fashion and climate allow.

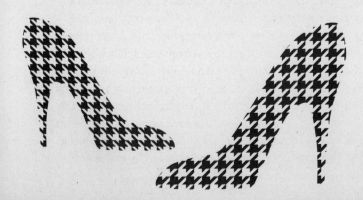

73 GO FOR LOW-KEY PRINTS

Have you ever entered a room – a party, perhaps, or a gathering of some sort – and had a stabbing feeling in your soul that people might think you've come in fancy dress? It's one of my personal dreads, and I have spent all my years in the fashion game trying to tiptoe the very thin line between looking enviably trend-aware, and going an inch too far and looking like the hired entertainment – a trumpet player, perhaps, in the samba band. Play it too safe, of course, and everyone will overlook your dress sense entirely and concentrate instead on other things you might be good at, such as whistling. Play it too wild and those same people will whisper about your fondness for galoshes the moment your back is turned.

It's a tricky balancing act – in fact, it's the very heart, the art, of fashion itself – and it's made all the more complicated when the fashion for 'mad prints' rolls around, as it does every fourth summer or so.

Mad prints are delightful, of course. I love them all . . . Those splashy florals which greet you like a slap in the eye with a flannel, the naive doodle prints, those blocky geometric ones that are very Pompidou Centre. All of them are crazy and cool. BUT they are all, without exception, teetering right on the brink when it comes to that line between incredibly wow and hopelessly whoops. And there's always the risk that you'll look like a sofa. Splashy prints take up twice the visual space of their more restrained cousins. They add weight. And they cause a kerfuffle. If people take one look at your outfit and say any of the following, you're in trouble:

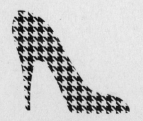

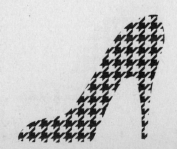

✳ 'Why have you come dressed as a pizza?'

✳ 'Very Habitat.'

✳ 'I had a cushion like that once.'

✳ 'Don't be mean, she's wearing it for a bet.'

✳ 'Whoah! You've spilled chicken casserole all down your front! Oh, you haven't? It's the new Vuitton print? Gosh, awfully sorry.'

If plumping for a print, then, here's what you need to know to avoid looking like a hot-air balloon:

✳ Dark backgrounds for a small, subtle print will shed weight (this has been dubbed the 'eight-pounds-lighter print').

✳ Big ethnic or graphic prints can disguise lumps and bumps (think tribal).

✳ While stripes of any variety are not flattering to an ample figure, geometric patterns and organic shapes are; they serve to break up the area covered, confusing the eye into believing it's smaller.

✳ Spriggy florals are, on the whole, kinder than wild, devil-may-care swirls. Laura Ashley was not wrong. Well, not *entirely* wrong.

✳ Keep your prints under control: a scarf (Pucci, Gucci or Hermès, perhaps) will confine your pattern in a nice contained space, like mint in a patio pot, rather than have it spill all over you like Japanese knotweed.

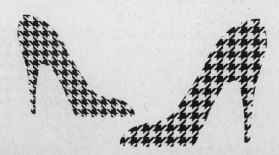

74 DISCRETION IS THE BETTER PART OF GLAMOUR, SO KEEP YOUR MIDRIFF UNDER WRAPS

I don't want to sound like a yowling old trout, but most naked midriffs are about as attractive as most naked bottoms. They loll over a waistband, like a neighbour over a fence. They bulge at the sides. They pucker at the back. Even though fashion has, strictly speaking, moved away from the mid section to focus on pastures new, they're still all over the place, littering the landscape like so many spare tyres. I saw one girl on the bus the other day and her midriff virtually had a life of its own; I half expected it to lean over and say, 'Nice weather we're having, don't you think?' or suggest an answer to nine across.

To my eye, even those rare toned tummies are mildly vulgar, a private place carelessly on parade. Ditto the small of the back, that low-rent lodging place for tramp-stamp tattoos. The fact is that a slim and stylish woman simply doesn't flash too much flesh, and even the flesh that is flashed needs to be treated judiciously. Take, for instance, the upper arm. That unassuming zone, which until now has meekly gone about the duty of joining your shoulder to your elbow, suddenly turns on you when you hit your mid thirties. Suddenly entire sections of your wardrobe are obsolete: the dinky tops, the tiny tees, the boob tubes, bra tops, camisoles and vests. Whole species, wiped out.

Some of us, of course, are more likely to go bingo than others. My fate, alas, is written in my genes, thanks to an Italian grandmother whose upper arms would swing jazzily in the breeze at summer picnics. I remember being hugged by those warm flannels of flesh, a place that smelled of security and lavender water and a peppermint lost in a handbag. Which is all very well if you're seventy-nine and have trouble remembering where you put your spectacles. At my age, when you're still considering a trip to Ibiza and have long glossy hair and good ankles (did I mention them?), well, slack triceps are nothing but a trial and a tribulation.

The solution lies in the cut of your tops. Sheer sleeves will mask chunky arms. Flippy sleeves on summer tops go a good way to distracting the eye while retaining adequate ventilation. Don't think, though, that you can divert attention from your wings by showing off your midriff. The world doesn't work like that.

'Most naked midriffs are about as attractive as most naked bottoms. They loll over a waistband, like a neighbour over a fence.'

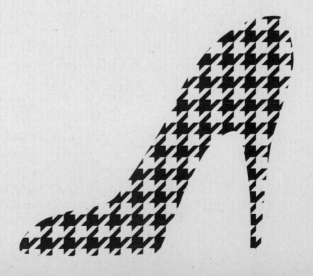

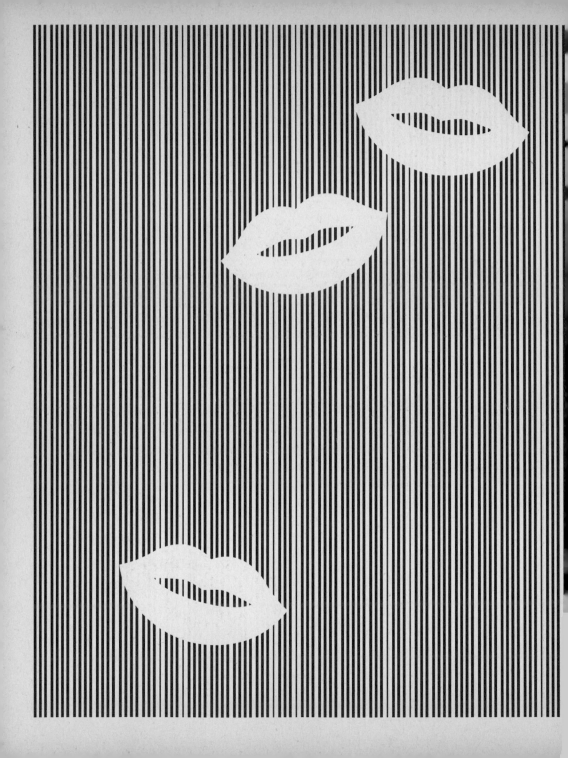

CHAPTER EIGHT
ON BEAUTY
How to Disguise Flab, Flubber, Blubber and Bloat

Most people, most of the time, are looking at your face. Promise. You may think that it is your grand mansion-block of a backside that is soaking up all of the attention, but more often than not, it is your eyes, your smile and your hands that will captivate an audience. Beyond all that, there are ways to buff up that body and make it work for you. All you need is the know-how.

75 MAINTAIN YOURSELF!

Style – though as much in the knowing as the doing – does require a certain degree of effort. Unless you are built like Cate Blanchett, or you're under the age of eighteen, you can't simply tumble out of bed and hope for the best in the belief that yesterday's make-up is somehow very Patti Smith circa 1978. You'll look more bush-backwards than bush baby.

So maximize your chances. Make the most of what you've got and you'll feel leagues better . . . Feel better and you'll look better. Simple, really. It's all about maintenance – not high, but constant, like a thermostat. Have your eyebrows professionally plucked. And grow your nails (stubby nails, stubby girl). Exfoliate! Exfoliate! See to cracked heels, cracked lips, grazes, bruises, calluses, rough skin and hair in inopportune places. One excruciatingly stylish woman of my acquaintance has a single nylon hair growing directly south from her otherwise pristine chin. It is possible she keeps it there for pure entertainment value, but, for me, that single hair quite ruins the undoubted power of her several Chanel jackets.

We all have our beauty bugbears, of course. Personally, I have learned to ignore my upper lip at my peril. Given that sporting facial hair of any description is an unparalleled faux pas in the protocols of femininity, I have entered into an agreement with several girlfriends that if we ever end up incapacitated and unable to wield a Tweezerman, we will visit each other at regular intervals to prune and bleach. This is staggering vanity, of course – but our fear is that without maintenance we could quite easily end up looking like Ben Stiller in *Dodgeball*. Our family and friends would flee the bedside in horror.

If similarly afflicted, you have a number of routes to redemption: you could thread (don't; it's grim), or wax, which makes you feel like a transsexual preparing for the Big Op. You could tweeze – which carries with it the old wife's threat that the chosen hair will return, bigger and stronger than before, like Popeye after a tin of spinach. Or there's always electrolysis. I can assure you from brute experience that this is precisely as painful as poking yourself in the eye with a sharp stick. 'There are more nerve endings per square inch here than on any other part of the body!' my therapist told me gaily as she inserted a very long needle into a follicle. 'There's only a minimal chance of scarring!' she added, zapping like mad while my eyes streamed and my nose ran all over her French manicure. These days, I find bleaching is best.

My argument here is that seemingly insubstantial things can kill a look at a glance. The devil, as any fashion editor will tell you if you ask politely, is not in Prada. It's in the detail. This is why a stylist rarely ventures out without a kit of canny essentials which will avert many a sartorial or cosmetic *crise*. Your emergency rations should, at the very least, include old-time favourites such as safety pins, dress-making pins, needle and thread. At home, keep spare buttons handy, together with nipple petals, stain-remover wipes, pumice, tweezers, a lint roller, Topstick double-stick tape (created for toupées but the tit-tape of choice for professional stylists). Carry a cottonwool bud or two for mascara spills, a tissue, a toothpick for spinach, a small mirror (to check for spinach). And at home, drape a silk scarf over your beautifully made-up face while you slip on your cashmere sweater. It's the least Elizabeth Taylor would have done in those heady old days.

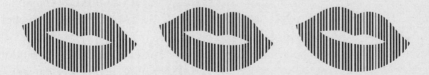

TAN YOURSELF **THIN**

By some fabulous trick of the light, a tan will shave off pounds, leaving you slender and toned without you even leaving your lounger. This is the fast-track to thin, but using the sun to do it is all wrong. A little lick of sun exposure is no bad thing (it is thought to combat depression and aid sleep); just don't overdo it. Instead of pegging yourself out in the midday sun, slathered in baby oil and reading John Grisham, go for one of the spectrum of tanning products on the market. Find what works for you. It may be airbrushing, bronzing mist, sunless foam, tanning gel, tinting mousse, sun-kissed moisturizer with SPF and a free toothbrush. Just don't risk UV exposure (that's A *and* B for those of you who aren't concentrating at the back). With all and any of these, the rule is to exfoliate first and wash hands afterwards. A gradual build-up will make you look less radioactive; don't go suddenly orange and surprise your friends by turning up to a barbecue looking like an Oompa-Loompa.

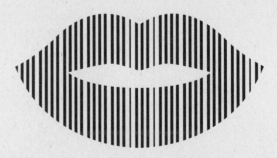

76 GET A HAIRSTYLE THAT WORKS WITH YOUR FACE, NOT THE FACE OF THAT GIRL IN THE MAGAZINE

Wanting to resemble our heroines is nothing new – women have always dreamed of having Audrey Hepburn's smile, or Marilyn Monroe's wiggle. But let this be a lesson to you: I once went to a hairdresser clutching a magazine picture of Jennifer Aniston and her Rachel cut (it was a while ago). I returned to the office and my boss said, 'Ooh, you've had a Lulu!' See? So many ways to fail.

According to celebrity hairdresser James Brown (the stylist who looks after Kate Moss), there are fat-busting ground rules for hair. 'Don't follow trends,' he says unequivocally. 'Hairstyles are not shoes – they won't look great on everyone.' And flatter your face – 'a square jaw needs a choppy cut below the chin, whereas round faces tend to suit a shoulder-length cut with a few layers'.

My own hairdresser, the redoubtable Jo Hansford of Mount Street in Mayfair (dubbed 'the best colourist on the planet' by US *Vogue*), knows the healing power of a great cut and colour. 'It takes the attention off the body and on to the face,' she says, adding:

✳ 'Make a round face longer by letting the hair grow to halfway down the neck. If you cut it to the jaw-line, you'll look like a pudding.'

✳ 'For long faces, try a fringe with a jaw-length bob; that way, you're effectively cutting the length of the face in half.'

✳ 'If your face is heart-shaped, use flick-ups to add width at the chin.'

And what of colour? If you tend to have pink-toned skin and high colour, Jo counsels caution. 'Stay away from warm tones – the golds and reds – because they'll make you look flushed. Go for cooler ash-browns, wheat-blondes, neutrals and caramels. And roots!' Yes? 'White roots make the hair look thin, they make you feel old and bald. They stop you being the best you can . . .'

Which is, after all, what this entire book is about. So get your grey done; it's not only ageing, it's disheartening. Personally, I always feel three pounds lighter when I leave Jo's salon with swishy, glossy, thoroughbred hair. (Not for long, though, since my favourite restaurant happens to be next door. Curses.)

77 LEARN HOW TO GIVE GOOD PHOTO

Generally speaking, I'm OK to look at. Not rosette-winning, you understand. But decent. I don't frighten kittens, and on a good day I scrub up well enough to garner an occasional compliment. Why is it, then, that photographs always make me look like Fiona in *Shrek*? I've got one holiday snap in which I'm the spit of Jeremy Paxman, so much so that people have started to ask why he was with us in a Menorcan tapas bar last summer. As one photo-phobic woman told *The Times* recently, 'From looking at our photographs, you'd think my husband was married to the au pair. If I died tomorrow, my children would hardly have a single photograph to remember me by.'

A survey by Hewlett Packard has found that two-thirds of us are 'deeply embarrassed' by many of our snaps. I'm with the majority on this one. I go from half-beauty to half-beast at the merest hint of flash. I always seem to be lurking on the periphery of any shot, red eyes ablaze, shirt askew, looking like Mrs Overall at a banquet. I have countless snaps where my nose – *just my nose* – has crept like a lone adventurer into the foreground, as if sniffing for attention. It has taken me years to work it out, but the truth is that, until fairly recently, I have been a hopeless subject. Someone only has to point a camera in my general direction and my face plays dead, my mouth forgets how to smile, my eyes start to lie and the wind blows in from the east to make my blouse billow out into the shape of a Mongolian yurt. When new photos appear, I scan them urgently for me, me, me, and I'm invariably gutted that the darling little nautical dress I was wearing has made me look like Georgie Porgie, having recently consumed both his pudding and his pie. In a world where image is all, where the air-brush is king and where I regularly have my photo taken doing interesting journalistic things, this is no party.

Dr David Lewis, a body-image expert and author of *Loving and Loathing, the Enigma of Personal Attraction*, has an explanation for this vexing state of affairs. We all apparently have three types of self-image: our 'real self' (how we believe ourselves to be), our 'other self' (how we believe other people regard us), and our 'ideal self' (the type of individual we most want to be). 'Our degree of liking or disliking snaps of ourselves depends on how closely they match not our real self, but our ideal self,' he says. 'A photo which, through careful lighting and camera angle, makes you appear closer to your ideal self will be treasured and preserved.'

Right then: how to seize one of these super-shots for yourself? Over the years, I have made a point of gathering tips from those in the know – the A-listers who are forever under the scavenger eye of the paparazzi lens, the models who only have to breathe to make the cover of *Vogue*, the photographers themselves who know precisely when to press the shutter and when to stop for tea. If you're forever de-tagging on Facebook, take a look at what I've learned, and what I will try to remember next time I'm on holiday (with or without Jeremy Paxman).

When photographed, try to:

✴ Turn slightly sideways, one foot forward à la Liz Hurley, weight on back foot. Stylist Charlotte Stockdale counsels thus: 'Stand three-quarters to the camera, shoulders back and smile with a closed mouth.'

✴ Lengthen neck, chin marginally down (think Linda Evangelista, not Yertle the Turtle). This tip ought to lessen a double chin. If it doesn't, try a polo-neck. Dropping the chin will also make your eyes appear bigger. I know, amazing isn't it? This is the Diana tilt, as you will recall from the *Panorama* interview.

✳ Station your arms fractionally away from the body to minimize the appearance of dinner-lady wings. 'You can,' says a fashion director at *Vogue*, 'create the illusion of slimmer arms by turning the arms outwards by your sides, so that the elbows are against your legs.' It's possible that you will look like a supplicating martyr in this pose – which is slimming, yes, but suspect on the beach in Ayia Napa.

✳ Shoulders back, abs in (but don't *suck* – you'll look as though you've just been slapped in the gut with a slipper).

✳ Look away from the camera just before the click, and then turn back. Ah, says your face, it's *you*! This trick will give your eyes a chance to look 'live' and you a reasonable chance of looking human.

✳ Tongue rests gently behind teeth, not glued to roof of mouth.

✳ Perfect your picture smile. If your mouth won't relax and behave, do a Keira Knightley: just put your lips together and blow gently. Christy Turlington was also adept at this soft pout. Clearly, it helps if you are unfeasibly beautiful, but we civilians can try it too. Don't try too hard or it will all go Louis Armstrong.

✳ Use your handbag to disguise your baggy bits. Grace Kelly did precisely this on the cover of *Life* magazine in 1956, when she shielded her baby bump with her Hermès handbag. So patrician! You can do it with a cardie slung over the shoulder, or a husband slung into the foreground. Grab a child or similar and station it in front of knock-knees, varicose veins, naff shoes, etc. (Though why you're wearing naff shoes is beyond me. Haven't you read Chapter Seven?)

✳ Place your gaze very slightly above the camera when the picture is taken. Jacqueline Kennedy apparently used this technique; it also helps reduce red eye.

✱ Sophie Dahl, a similarly dab hand at the flattering photo, says, 'Don't chatter – you'll have your mouth open in the pictures and you'll look like a freak.' If you possess a particularly animated face, as I do, settle it or you'll look like a gargoyle.

✱ Avoid white dresses – they'll make you bigger, flatter, fatter. Yes, even the bride. Quite why the Victorians obliged a woman to wear white on the most important day of her young life is beyond me. If concerned on your big day, perhaps use bridesmaids, ushers and sundry floral arrangements by way of disguise (see above). An ivory or coffee tone is generally kinder than end-of-spectrum white.

✱ Don't squint into the sun. Wear shades. Or look the other way.

✱ If Desperate No 1: play with your hair. Diane von Furstenberg has been doing this in photos for decades and it takes years off her, making her look coltish and adorable, like a foal.

✱ If Desperate No 2: look back over your shoulder towards the camera. Why do you think they're always doing that in the Boden catalogue?

✱ Find a photographer who loves you. Mario Testino, perhaps, whose life's work it is to make women look beautiful. If Mario is booked, at least find someone who cares enough to make sure there isn't a flagpole sprouting out of your head.

✱ Once you've found a photographer who loves you (hey, no pressure, but it would be great if it was your partner, for convenience if nothing else), you now need to give them the heads up on lighting. It's a girl's best friend and a woman's redeeming saviour. Aim for a flattering light to give a softening, wrinkle-smoothing effect, rather than a harsh light which threatens to create nasty nose shadows or badger eyes. Play about with the lighting, know where the sun is, consider background colours. It may be a bit much for a quick snap, but it is worth understanding a little about light if you want to give yourself the best possible chance of a decent portrait. After all, it's going to be on your mother's mantelpiece for decades to come.

✷ Get your photographer to tilt the camera upwards a smidge for a more flattering angle: it will elongate the face and improve your proportions.

✷ Always remember that photographs don't tell the whole truth. They are not a mirror image, so you're bound to be thrown by an unfamiliar version of your own face. According to psychologist Linda Papadopoulos, 'Photographs aren't very representative of what we look like in reality . . . [they're] just a record of one static moment. People are never completely still like they are in a photograph, and animation changes the way we look. In studies, people are often rated as significantly better-looking in person than in photographs, and that's because of personal qualities, such as confidence.' This, I like.

✷ One more lighting tip: if you want sincere flattery, don't wait for your partner to come up with the goods. Do it yourself with tea lights. Or a collection of church pillar candles installed on the coffee table as if waiting for a treble chorister to sing 'O for the Wings of a Dove'. According to director of photography Adam Hall, 'Candlelight is very warm, very soft and irons out wrinkles and imperfections.' Perfect, particularly for romantic assignations, cosy suppers, a girls' get-together. We're not, though, living in Dickensian London, so for everyday purposes invest in superior lighting for your home. This is your space! It should work for you. Proper lighting, by which I mean plenty of choice from floor and table lamps with warm-coloured shades, up-lighters to bounce light off the walls, a hanging light with a wide shade pulled low over a dining table – will be so much kinder than an overhead strip, the kind of light that beats you up and leaves you for dead. Save that for your bathroom, where honesty trumps artifice every time.

✷ Finally, don't run scared of the camera or you'll end up with vast tracts of your life uncharted, the you of your youth lost forever. Besides, when you look at old photos that you once hated because you looked fat and old and gormless . . . what do you see now? Not so bad after all, right?

IF MAGAZINES CHEAT,
THEN YOU CAN TOO

Remind yourself, as you say 'cheese' and hope for the best, that the images which surround us are pure untrammelled fantasy. As supermodel Christy Turlington explains, 'Advertising is so manipulative. There's not one picture in magazines today that's not air-brushed. It's funny – when women see pictures of models in fashion magazines and say, "I can never look like that", what they don't realize is that no one can look that good without the help of a computer.' Or, as Cindy Crawford sums up, 'I think women see me on the cover of magazines and think that I never have a pimple or bags under my eyes. You have to realize that's after two hours of hair and make-up, plus retouching. Even I don't wake up looking like Cindy Crawford.'

Lately, the kind of air-brushing and retouching usually reserved for top models (who, heaven knows, are the last women who need it) has become available to the masses. Snappy Snaps, for example, has an air-brushing service for customers who want to enhance their holiday snaps without all the bother of a beauty overhaul. You can brighten dark circles, lengthen legs, erase jelly roll, whiten teeth, just like they do in the art departments of magazines. If you want a deeper clean, retouchphoto.co.uk can give you a complete picture facelift, eliminating saggy jowls, eye-bags and unprepossessing husbands. The only thing you can't do is cut-and-paste an Adonis in a thong to stand at your side. Actually, hang on a mo . . . you *can* have an Adonis! There you go: the world's perfect picture.

Alternatively, cut out the middle man and do it at source. You can now buy digital cameras with a 'slimming feature' which stretches your image, visually removing about ten pounds in the process. It's called 'digital dieting'. Useful for internet brides.

TREAT BEAUTY PROMISES WITH CALCULATED CAUTION

There are certain bitter truths that the beauty industry and all its pretty messengers don't want you to uncover, partly because it would put them out of a job, but chiefly because it would forever pop the bubble of sweet-smelling hope that informs the whole expensive endeavour. So get with the programme. Know, for instance, that models who look thin enough to have eating disorders usually have eating disorders. Know that time will indeed bestow fine lines upon your brow, and hypo-poxy-nutrino-placenta-extract in a costly porcelain jar will do little to help. Know, above all, that rubbing cream on your bottom will not shrink it.

Enticing as they seem, with their promises of smoothing, polishing and encouragement of lypolysis, cellulite creams are not going to do much more than exercise your credit card. You'd be better off rubbing yourself down with lemon curd. Save your money in a little pot – perhaps that empty porcelain jar – and spend it on a rowing machine. Now, take a deep breath and wise up to your worst fears. Extract your head from beneath the duvet of deception and take a good look at your thighs. If there's cellulite there, get a grip and tackle it.

DON'T GO FOR THE SELL –
GO FOR THE CELLULITE

Laser energy, vacuum massage, micro-encapsulated caffeine tights, infra-red light, guarana soap, jeans infused with retinol serum, radio-frequency, crossed fingers, liposuction ... The incredible choice of everyday miracles available to the poor woman afflicted with cellulite points up quite what a persistent and universal problem it is. In 2007, a full 85 per cent of American women were lumbered with the stuff, which is one heck of a lot of women walking out of their bedrooms backwards. This vast expanse of orange peel is undoubtedly a serious worry for a serious number of women. Cellulite is, alas, predominantly a girl thing, its formation closely linked to female sex hormones, which is why, as a rule, men have no need for infra-red pants.

As anyone who's got it knows, cellulite is formed as fat cells enlarge with age. The bastards. They nudge up against connecting fibres, a bit like a balloon being blown up through a string vest (one of those delightful images we could really do without). What you see on the surface is a characteristic dimple effect, which sounds cute. Cellulite is not cute. It is a curse. So zap it. Stop thinking 'wonder fix'; start thinking 'Wonder if I can fix this?' Stop tinkering about with your exterior, and start work on your interior. I know it may not be quite as thrilling as buying a lovely bottle of goo in a pretty pink box. But this little lot will work. In time.

✱ **Eat well**. Embrace plenty of vegetation, fruit and whole grains, while introducing a moratorium on processed food, sugar, alcohol and caffeine. Some time ago, I remember reading the brilliantly titled *Cellulite My Arse!* (Vermilion), in which author Shonagh Walker recommended the consumption of foods that stimulate the detoxing process, such as celery, cucumber, leeks and onion. Worth a try.

✱ **Hydrate**. Drink lots. Water, not coffee, not juice, not Merlot. The idea is to sluice.

✱ **Exercise**. To stimulate circulation; get up off your bottom. Show it to the world, not just to a cushion cover.

✱ **Don't smoke**.

✱ **Slash salt**. It encourages fluid retention.

✱ **Go organic** – to reduce your unintentional intake of oestrogen and other hormones lurking in mass-produced meat.

✱ **Body brush**. Work upwards with a dry natural-bristled brush while humming to yourself (bathroom acoustics are always great, aren't they?).

✱ **Massage**. A lymphatic drainage massage may well help to stimulate that sluggish circulation. Even if it doesn't, it's a fine way to spend a lunch hour.

✱ **Self-tan**. Cellulite is much less obvious on darker skin.

79 DO A DIANA AND GET A COLONIC

So, you're feeling sallow, baggy, gassy and bloated? You always get standing space on the Tube? Your hair and skin is limp and your tongue an interesting shade of beige? It's alimentary, my dear reader. You ought to give some thought to your internal flora. I know it's not exactly dinner-party conversation (unless you're German), but what goes on down there can have a significant impact on how good you look in a bikini. Chew on the fact that our distinctly unnatural modern diet does our internal ecology few favours; over-processed food, high-fructose corn syrup, antibiotics, great slabs of meat . . . these things arrive in the gut and subtly upset the balance, like an ex at a wedding.

There are ways to improve your equilibrium. Bran, psyllium or ispaghula husk and natural live yoghurt are all good places to start. Heidi Klum recommends bathing in Epsom Salts to reduce bloating; I recommend that you don't drink through a straw. If it's just a little local difficulty, the Gut Trust advocates probiotics – those kindly bacteria that reside in small yoghurt drinks or (better still) in acidophilus capsules – together with plenty of hydration and not too much prawn Madras.

If things really have seized up, you could always give colonic irrigation a whirl. You'd be in good company. Princess Diana made thrice-weekly pilgrimages to London's Hale Clinic where she underwent what fast became known as the Royal Flush. It was also a favoured technique of John Lennon, and of Mae West, who apparently started every day with a refreshing morning enema. 'I'm sure,' said her nutritionist Bernard Jensen, 'that this simple practice greatly contributed to her unusual vitality, bright-mindedness and long-lasting attractiveness, as true beauty is but a reflection of the beauty within.' Ah, true enough, Bernard, true enough. Today, Kim Basinger, Goldie Hawn and Demi Moore are said to be fans of irrigation, while Courtney Love swears by it. As she recently told *Harper's Bazaar* magazine: 'They really did the trick for me . . . I hate reading magazines where the actresses are saying, "Broccoli and fish, broccoli and fish." You liars!'

If you do take the plunge, you'll find that a colonic *lavage* (as it is called in refined circles) is not nearly as dreadful as you might expect; I found it all very gung-ho and far less embarrassing than I'd anticipated, a bit like childbirth or karaoke (though significantly less painful than both). Weight loss, though by no means its primary function, may be a welcome spin-off.

THE BEAUTY BREAKFAST

When you're weary, feeling small, what you really need is this energy-boosting, body-buffing breakfast. It promises to aid digestion and elimination, leaving you with beautiful clear skin and bundles of get-up-and-go. Here's what to do:

✳ Before you go to bed, take a tub of live yoghurt.

✳ Mix it with fruit juice or water to give it the consistency of a shake.

✳ Add a handful of jumbo porridge oats, some seeds (linseeds, sunflower seeds, flaxseeds), plus chopped prunes, chopped apricots, chopped dates, chopped almonds.

✳ Leave in the fridge overnight to ferment.

✳ Eat in the morning.

✳ Feel lovely.

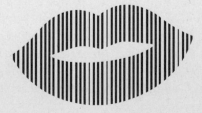

80 LEARN TO USE BLUSHER PROPERLY

I have a face shaped, broadly, like a side plate. A generous observer might remark that it's more heart-shaped, but even a kindly soul would admit that I don't appear to have much in the way of cheekbones. I've always really fancied one of those wicked, chiselled faces that can grate cheese, stop traffic and fell men at a single stroke. Wouldn't we all? Well, anything's possible.

If you spend any time at all in the company of models, you'll soon notice that a potent alchemy goes on backstage at a fashion shoot or show. Pretty-ish girls with pasty faces, moon faces, pie faces turn up – and later (often much later) they emerge with the visage of Venus. They have been chiselled by Rodin, they are muse, they are grace, they are siren. They have been lent high cheekbones and defined jaw-lines. They are slim of nose and long of neck. And it's all been achieved with the skilful application of cosmetics.

Clearly, most of us have more pressing engagements in our day than walking to the end of a runway and back, ad infinitum or until someone lights us a Marlboro and tells us to stop – but many of the techniques known to the make-up gurus are well worth learning. They won't change your face completely, of course. You won't catch sight of yourself and think, 'Ooh, hello Angelina!' But the judicious use of the principles of contouring will be yet another arrow in your quiver of weight-loss techniques, right up there with small plates and magic pants.

To get the low-down (and the highlights) of contouring, I paid a visit to Terry Barber, a master in the art and creative director at Mac Cosmetics, the foremost international make-up brand for such endeavours.

Me: What is contouring?
TB: The art of contouring is the true art of make-up. Make-up itself was originally designed to accentuate the structure of a face rather than to decorate it. It's all about light, really. Darker colours

will cause an area of the face to recede, while lighter colours will bring it out. You see the techniques most clearly on film and stage, but it's all about the trickery of make-up and it's something that can easily be adapted for everyday life if you know how. As a make-up artist, I've seen that what makes women really tick is when you give them a cheekbone, better still if the method is undetectable. Eyes and lips come and go, they're trends, but make-up which enhances bone structure will be with us for ever.

Me: Who taught you how to do it?

TB: I learned contouring from Liza Minnelli, who virtually worked in black and white. She'd put a little black under her jaw and cheekbone, and then blend it all the way up into the hairline, using the curl of her hair to accentuate the cheek. She would paint on a face, drawing on downward eyes – the 'Halston Face'; she'd flick the contour up into the apple of the cheek and highlight the centre of her chin and the T-bar of her face in white. It was pure showbiz.

Me: Anyone else?

TB: Yep. Linda Evangelista taught me a lot about contouring too. She'd put a flick of dark brown under the chin to separate the face from the neck. But then, she lived on camera ...

Me: Should we all be putting dark-brown flicks on our chins? Wouldn't it look like a goatee?

TB: Products have changed so much lately, so it's much more subtle. I remember in the eighties, when it was all New Romantic, you'd have white skin and use grey to contour. You'd end up with stripes ramped across your face. Now, though, pigments are jet-milled, really fine, with mineralized formulas. These products 'pop' the skin and don't look like a mask.

Me: OK, so how do you do it?

TB: Here's how ...

Shading: Contour products are meant to look like skin, so you see lots of taupes, beiges, ivories, flesh tones, darker skin tones – which can appear broadly similar to the untrained eye. Use a contour formula, such as Mac's Sculpt, to shade and give depth under a cheekbone, to narrow a temple or heart-shaped jaw-line.

225

Go for a tobacco colour that gives shade. But you don't want a dark-brown jaw-line, so blend and play – always in good light, try for even daylight if possible. Dust through the edge of the face.

Here's a foolproof trick for cheek contouring: imagine a line (or hold a pencil) between the top of the ear and the corner of the lip. Shade that line. Imagine another line from the corner of the lip to the outer corner of the eye. Shading shouldn't come in further than that. If your face is wide, slim it down by applying contour colour to the outer jaw-line; a darker shade below the jaw will make it more distinct. Like this . . .

Me: Ooh, yes, that works! Should I use blusher too?

TB: Yes.

Me: How?

TB: The idea is to make your cheekbones look 3D. Use a cream or gel blusher and go up into the hairline. If you want, you can go beyond your usual contours to accentuate further than the natural shadow. Then you need to . . .

Highlight: Use ivory or a clear, glisten product for accentuating the 'crest' areas where light hits the face. Add a little cream highlight to the top of the cheekbone and the brow bone.

Eyes: Highlight the inner corner of the eye socket to the bridge of the nose, right in that pocket of shadow. Think Chanel! I call it 'drawn-on surgery'.

Nose: I wouldn't bother with nose contouring – it's a video technique. Leave it to Naomi. If you want to, just powder the sides of the nose to take off any shine (which widens the nose). We're talking about light, really, so leave the bridge of the nose unpowdered to give the illusion of narrowness.

Me: Brilliant. I have cheekbones! I have never had cheekbones. I think I might cry. Etc.

For similar hands-on advice, book in for a one-to-one session at a Mac Counter – at one of their stand-alone shops, or in any large department store. Ask for a member of the Pro team, who will have worked on fashion shoots and behind the scenes at runway shows; they'll know exactly how to release your thinner self.

NO-OW BROW KNOW-HOW

You have the ultimate face-shapers right there. Your eyebrows. So get them to work on your behalf. I'm not expecting the full Fiona Bruce, but a little lift here, a lengthen there, can have a dramatic impact on a pudding face. Go pro if you can. If not, a Tweezerman is your best weapon. Pluck after a shower, once your pores are warm and forgiving, and use a bright, inquisitive light. Get those stray mid-brow hairs first, then pluck away *beneath* the brow, working towards a coquette's arch at a point which feels right for you. Terry Barber has the following tips: 'Feather in the eyebrow with a pencil, using delicate strokes to elongate it by one or two hairs. The inner corners of the eyebrow shouldn't hook down too much – it makes the nose wider. Marilyn Monroe's sleepy glamour had a lot to do with those eyebrows. They were quite wide apart, with an arch directly above the pupil. It was all very architectural . . . You can measure the ideal eyebrow by holding the pencil upright from the side of the nose to the brow. That's where your brows should start. Any closer and your nose will start to look wider.'

Then brush your brows north with an old toothbrush, and trim unruly ones with a pair of baby scissors. If your eyebrows are scant, use powder eyeshadow in the appropriate colour to fill in the gaps, working in a light feathery motion. Very pale eyebrows, or grey brows, may need tinting. If they are really sparse, an expert will be able to tattoo them in (go to as smart a salon as you can afford; this is not an area for economy). You can, of course, go too far with this. If you ever get to the stage where you are drawing on your own eyebrows in marmalade-coloured pencil, you'll know it's time to put that mirror away.

CHAPTER NINE
MAKE A DATE WITH YOUR METABOLIC RATE
Where Exercise Fits In

We all know the original fat-busting equation: to lose weight, you need to eat less or move more. It's all down to the laws of thermodynamics. Fine, you can tinker around with pills and potions, ointments, unguents and self-help audio tapes. But if you want to succeed, you're going to need to stir yourself. Just a bit. Fairly often. The best way to get going is to introduce moderate cardiovascular exercise into your daily life. Don't book it into your diary as a special occasion; modify your lifestyle just a modicum and you'll see the difference next time you're stuck in a changing cubicle with only a wraparound mirror for company.

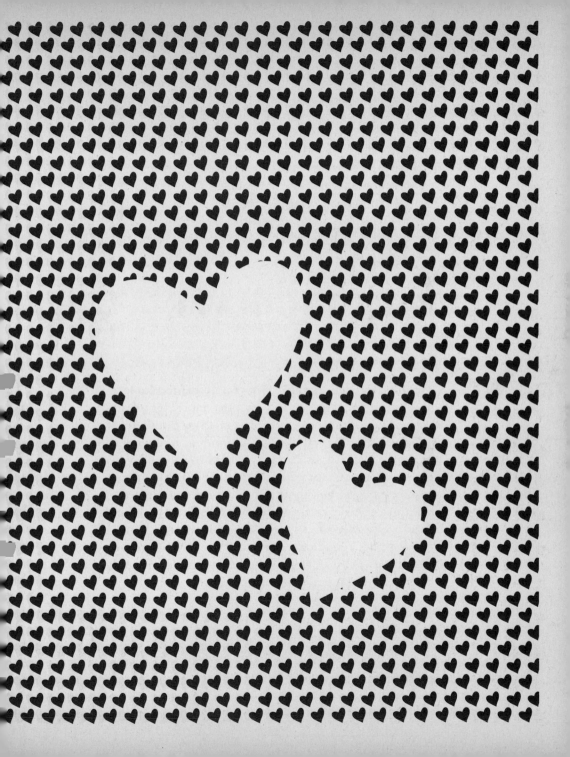

81 GET BUSY

There's a revealing scene in *Ab Fab* when the dissolute Edina decides it's high time she should shift some weight. Daughter Saffy, in typically sensible mode, says, 'Look, Mum, all you've got to do is eat less and take a bit of exercise.' Edina bites back, 'Sweetie, if it was that easy, everyone would be doing it.'

The problem is that most of us aren't. A rather dispiriting survey by a skincare company not long ago found that we spend 14 hours and 28 minutes a day taking the weight off our feet – the equivalent of 36 years of our adult lives sitting down. Allowing for eight hours' sleep, we spend a meagre hour and a half on our feet, active, each day.

Yet we humans aren't programmed to sit, sit, sit. Physiologically speaking, we haven't changed a great deal from our days of roaming the great savannah in search of prey. We're designed to walk many miles a day, not cosy up to a computer screen with a box of iced buns and a crick in the neck. So stand up, right now. Do something about it. Get in touch with your ancient self! Activity not only burns calories, builds muscle mass and raises your base metabolic rate; it will also keep you out of the fridge.

Exercise, if you're not already a fan, really needs to be something that you can weave into your life, not something you do as a grand gesture, expecting bunting and applause on your return. Do it in regular bursts rather than great blistering chunks.

The buzzword here is integrative exercise – which is a natty way of saying 'move around a bit more'. Studies show that several five-to ten-minute bouts of activity throughout a day will promote cardiovascular and respiratory health, lower your risk of diabetes and improve your longevity. Start small. A brisk walk. A run down the road. A run back. Reach a new lamp-post every day. Don't expect a medal (unless you have just run a marathon, in which case, congratulations, it's all yours). But watch out: studies have shown that you're likely to pile up your plate if you've done even moderate exercise. So try not to see a run around the block as an excuse to eat four crumpets as soon as you're back in the comfort of your own kitchen. Yes, you deserve a high-five, but not a high-calorie carbo feast which leaves butter smeared on your chin.

Here, then, are a few tips on how to thintegrate:

✳ **Use the stairs, No 1**. Spurn the lift; cultivate claustrophobia; develop an unfounded fear of escalators. 'Using the stairs is not seen as normal,' says Amelia Lake, a research fellow in clinical medical science at Newcastle University. 'In most [new] buildings it's very difficult to find a staircase. The focal point when you enter tends to be the lift. In certain buildings, you'll even find that using the stairs will set off the fire alarm.' Architect Will Alsop takes a stronger line: 'If you really wanted to do something about [the obesity crisis],' he says, 'you could take all the elevators out of all the buildings in London. Then people would be fit.' He's right. When employees of the University Hospital of Geneva were banned from using the lift for twelve weeks – a move which increased their daily climb from five to twenty-three flights of stairs – their aerobic capacity increased by an average of 8.6 per cent and their body fat levels fell by 2 per cent.

✳ **Find a way to enjoy walking more**. Fill your iPod with tunes. Hum. Snoop into people's front rooms, join Neighbourhood Watch, take up the lost art of perambulation in the park, perhaps wearing a feathered picture hat. As you march, listen to stirring opera, or do as Stephen Fry did and take your dynamic daily constitutional accompanied by an audiobook of Rufus Sewell reading Ian Fleming: 'You don't notice you're walking,' reports Fry, 'and you walk faster and faster because it's all very tense.'

✳ **If you're into gadgets, get yourself a pedometer** (one of those machines that counts the steps you take). According to scientists at Stanford University, having a daily goal is an important predictor of increased physical activity. A review recently showed that pedometer use is associated with significant increases in physical activity and decreases in BMI and blood pressure. Who cares if it makes you look nerdy? Better a fit nerd than a fat sack.

✷**Discover pole-dancing**; consider belly-dancing; take up tap . . . or just dance around the room. Whatever. Do it for ten minutes a day, or every time you're waiting for the kettle to boil. Choose your dance routine with care. If you take up swing, it'll cost you 372 calories an hour (especially if you do the East Coast Lindy Hop); belly-dancing burns 378; salsa 372; and ballroom 216 calories an hour (more if you do it in full make-up, silver stilettos and a big swishy skirt).

✷**Get off the bus one stop early**. Yes, I know you've heard it before, but have you ever done it? Do you even take the bus? If not, this one won't work for you. But if you do, run behind that bus and try to catch up, imagining that you have left your BlackBerry or your birth-control pills on the back seat. If you take the Tube, alight at an earlier station and take in the view. Walk the rest of the way, looking upwards to allow your gaze to rest on architecture you've never noticed before. Change your perspective.

✷**Spring clean**. Commune with your inner control freak. Vacuum for fifteen minutes and you've killed fifty-eight calories.

✷**Walk the kids to school**. Hey, it's better for them too, so you're spreading the love. If you have no kids, walk someone else's kids to school (ask first).

✷**Do one wild thing**. Abandon yourself. Get intense. Lose it on the dance floor.

✷**Develop an interest in something arcane and hard to find**. Like ammonites. Go out and find your holy grail.

✷**Bid for a bike on eBay** and cycle to work.

✷**Forage for your lunch**. Wild foods are nutritious, leafy and free, and you get to walk through meadows with a purpose (without having to play golf).

✷**Use the stairs, No 2**. Instead of piling shoes and shampoo and Lego on the bottom stair so you can take everything upstairs in one go, take things one at a time.

✴ **Stand up!** Standing burns thirty-six more calories per hour than sitting.

✴ **Indulge in impromptu games**. Play tag, stick-in-the-mud, basketball. You'll burn a hundred calories in ten minutes and your kids will still want to talk to you when they hit puberty.

✴ **Consider getting a dog**. Energetic walking is known to be the single most valuable integrative exercise you can do, and an inquisitive terrier is as energetic a beast as walks the earth. I borrowed Rhubarb the Patterdale terrier from a friend a few months back and my rather stagnant life was transformed as I was whizzed across the park each morning. If you're single, a cool dog has the added bonus of being fantastic man-bait. Weimaraners and puppies work best.

✴ **Join a rambling club**, or . . .

✴ **Indulge in speed shopping**, or . . .

✴ **Post letters one at a time**, or . . .

✴ **Chi walk**. This involves meditating as you walk, focusing on muscles and movement; its exponents promise that you'll get fitter – and slimmer – faster. You might also become a better person. Just think!

✴ **Drink more water**. You'll *have* to get up to go to the bathroom. Visit the one up three flights of stairs, not the one at the end of the corridor.

✴ **Lose the remote**. If elderly, keep forgetting where you left your teeth; if younger, your mobile phone.

✴ **Move from the 'burbs**. A study of 200,000 Americans at Rutgers University in New Jersey found that city dwellers were on average six pounds lighter than their suburban counterparts, largely because, instead of driving, they walk more. 'In very dense urban environments, you get local shops and facilities mixed up together,' says Tim Townshend, a Newcastle academic and former town planner. 'There's an awful lot more walking involved, just because of the inconvenience of driving.' Interestingly, then, city living creates what is known as the 'eco-slob' effect, where the healthy, environmentally friendly option also happens to be the path of least resistance. By contrast, if your life is all mall and sprawl, you're more likely to travel by car and lay down the lard. This – together with the greater prevalence of gyms and lipo and bitchy girlfriends – explains why New Yorkers are slimmer than Americans as a whole.

✳ **If you are 'burb-bound, try 'Mallercise'.** This is the craze for power-walking while window-shopping (shoe manufacturers now market 'mall-walker' shoes featuring 'extra traction for smoother, slicker mall floors'). On the plus side, mall-walking is traffic-free, rain-resistant and relatively safe; it can burn two hundred calories in half an hour, if you include the odd lunge and you laugh in the face of the escalator. On the down side, you may spot a lust-have pair of ankle boots in Kurt Geiger or a must-have cookie in the Dough Shop. Either way, bang goes the benefit.

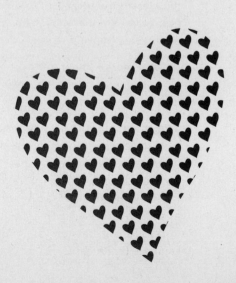

82 FIND YOUR THING AND STICK WITH IT

According to received wisdom, in order to lose one pound of fat, you must burn or dodge 3,600 calories. Received wisdom can be so depressing, can't it? Well, fret not. Don't think lifetime, think lunchtime. Start now. A little jog. A step class for beginners. A cycle to work. Roller-disco. You choose.

If you have a wandering attention span and pathetic stamina (*Moi aussi!*), you perhaps need a goal. Before my wedding, for instance, plagued by the prospect of a small, backless white dress scattered with hand-sewn seed pearls, I somehow managed a session with a personal trainer three mornings a week for a year. And when I say mornings, I mean freakishly early, Anna Wintour early. We'd meet before six, work out for an hour and I'd be showered, dressed and in the office by seven fifteen. OK, so sometimes I didn't shower, but I *always* dressed.

Children change all that, of course. These days, I'm still up at the crack, but I spend those early hours searching high and low for a missing shoe or stirring porridge or trying to get satsuma juice out of the sofa cushions. In my more benevolent moments, I convince myself that all this rushing about is the rough equivalent of paying someone thirty pounds an hour to put me through my paces on a cross-trainer and then count while I perform two hundred expert crunches. Not so. It's cheaper, yes, but nowhere near as effective.

Here is the bullet you need to bite: proper exercise requires an element of planning, space-making and commitment. You have to persevere. Tone was not built in a day. As an added incentive, it's worth noting that studies have found that the less muscle you possess, the harder it is to lose weight (because muscle is metabolically active, whereas body fat is inactive – as anyone furnished with a sizeable, sleepy rump well knows).

If you are obstinately vain, you'll also need to develop a carapace that means you don't care what you look like when exercising. I'd like to say that I don't give a monkey's, but I've always found that exercising is a peculiarly intimate thing to do in public – a bit like speaking French or breastfeeding. I abhor sweating in front of strangers and will go to great lengths to avoid physical activity of any kind if it has to be done in a crowd. For this reason, my gym kit really matters, perhaps more than any other outfit in my life. So I wear amazing stretchy, hold-you-in track-pants by a very right-on yoga label called Prana. I like to think I look very slightly Cindy Crawford in a dim light (this is gym psych, people, and it counts).

The real poke in the eye is that most gyms are inhabited by a handful of jaw-drop women who really *do* look like Cindy Crawford, even in a very bright light. My advice is to ignore them. Ignore their bouncy ponytails and their pert buttocks. Ignore their terry hot pants and their foxy tops. Concentrate on your mission. Hum if necessary. If time and commitment are issues, it pays to be choosy. Rather than go at it like a banshee in a turret, decide which part of your body needs most attention and target it:

✻ **Yoga** will give you a strong torso (from the abdominal work required to maintain those balancing postures) and muscular definition in the arms (if you stay long enough in downward dog). Muscles are lengthened through stretching, so regular yoga should leave you with a longer, leaner body. It also aids posture. Some yogas are more dynamic and demanding than others. Regular Bikram or Astanga will clearly be more beneficial than lying down in a room that smells of patchouli while chanting Om through your third eye.

✻ **Running** promises enhanced muscle definition and lower body fat, particularly if you go long distance. Beware shin splints and jogger's nipple (also known as raver's nipple, bloody mary nipple, weightlifter's nipple and gardener's nipple. Though one suspects you'd have to garden freakishly hard to do any real damage).

✻ **Walking**, like climbing stairs, should perk up your buttocks. 'Walkers,' says exercise expert Joanna Hall, 'can have great buttocks as, unlike recreational jogging, with each stride the hip fully extends, targeting the gluteal muscles of the bottom, creating a firm, shapely and uplifted posterior.' Set a smart pace (see how over the page), and keep those abs in. According to Hall, 'the latest abdominal research suggests that training the abdominals in an upright position, as one ought to when walking with good technique, is more effective than using traditional sit-ups as it builds the muscle in a functional way, doing something the body was designed to do'.

✴ **Swimming** is a superlative all-round workout and will give you a defined waist and strong shoulders, together with toned pecs. If you are blonde, it might also turn your hair green. And verrucas are a constant threat. But don't let me put you off.

✴ **Pilates** will deftly streamline a body, the series of strengthening movements imbuing you with elegance rather than hard body-tone. You'll gain spine mobility and core strength, together with good alignment, which will make you an altogether more efficient beast, and all without breaking into a sweat. Little wonder that an estimated twelve million people around the world practise it. Says its originator, Ron Fletcher: 'People mistake it for an exercise regimen, and it's not. It's an art and it's a science and it's a study of movement . . . you think about what you're doing.' Using a reformer will isolate muscle groups for greater efficacy, though you may feel as though you're trapped inside a slide rule.

'Regular Bikram or Astanga will clearly be more beneficial than lying down in a room that smells of patchouli while chanting Om through your third eye.'

Exercise of any description is a potent mood-enhancer, as you'll notice if you compare the faces going into the gym with the ones coming out. Cardiovascular activity can escort you from the doldrums to the crest of a wave in a mere twenty minutes, its benefits being not only physiological but psychological too. You know you're doing yourself good, which is a real pat on the back; there's nothing like a well-used sneaker to put a spring in your step.

If you exercise in a concerted way for an extended period, you may even encounter the fabled glory that is an endorphin rush. Endorphins are produced by your pituitary gland and hypothalamus in response to strenuous exercise, excitement or orgasm. They have a similar effect to opiates, in that they can relieve pain and bestow a pleasing sense of well-being and even euphoria.

Personally, I have felt many things during heavy exercise (hot, bothered, fatigued, angry, peevish, bored, a throbbing sensation in my left knee), but never euphoria. The conclusion I draw from this unscientific and selective study of myself is that I'm not exercising long or hard enough. If you do, however, it's possible that you too could experience a runner's high, and the point of enduring the undoubted hell of the London Marathon in the April sleet will suddenly, blissfully, become known to you. All power, I say. Though the very existence of this exercise buzz has been questioned ever since the idea was first propagated in the seventies, German scientists have recently used PET scans and other technical wizardry to show that the limbic and prefrontal areas of a runner's brain (those associated with emotions) are indeed affected by the release of endorphins following a two-hour run.

HOW TO WALK OFF THE WEIGHT

'Walking is potentially the most effective and accessible form of body-toning exercise,' says fitness and diet expert Joanna Hall. 'You can definitely walk fit, walk firm and walk off weight. Technique and pace are crucial for best results. On my twenty-eight-day "walk off weight" programme [find out more on joannahall.com], we have people walking off ten pounds and ten inches in just four weeks! Do it right and it definitely works. Here's how:

First establish your **optimum walking pace**:

✴ Start to walk, progressively increasing your pace every thirty seconds (speeding up your arm-swing really helps), until you are just about to break into a jog. This is your break-point walking pace.

✴ Ease back off this pace by 5 to 10 per cent, and you have your optimum walking pace.'

So, no slouching, no lolloping, no foot-dragging. No pigeon toes, no stopping for a fag or a muffin. If you're really going to walk your weight off, you need to do it with conviction (though that curious hip-rolling which long-distance competitive walkers engage in is probably a technique too far). Settle for something that feels like exercise rather than a stroll, with a quicker heartbeat and a bit of colour in your cheeks. Aim to do it three or four times a week, for as long as it takes to play an entire CD on your iPod. And, though walking in high heels is both an art and a sport, do wear properly fitted, springy trainers if you want to walk fit. Doing it in Gucci sling-backs will do you no good at all. Probably the only example of human endeavour in which this is the case.

83 WEAN YOURSELF OFF YOUR FAVOURITE SOAP

Research has shown that Britons are consuming 20 per cent fewer calories on average than in the seventies. But our level of physical activity has plummeted even more sharply. We live in what experts call 'an obesogenic environment' – a world which lends itself, inexorably, to the accretion of fat. For a potted version of our fantastically busy, woefully lazy lives, consider the following snippets of data: only 20 per cent of men and 10 per cent of women are now employed in active occupations; chores such as washing and cleaning are increasingly mechanized (electric toilet brush, anyone?); television-viewing has more than doubled from thirteen hours per week in the sixties; more than 80 per cent of people would avoid a two-mile walk . . . As a result, we are increasingly a doughnut-based life-form. And the striking thing about doughnuts? They don't move very fast.

If we'd care to admit it, most of us are prone to a pathological inertia. To do anything beyond breathing, sleeping and snuffling through the contents of the fridge, we need a gentle push. Some of us may need a kick in the rump.

And the first hurdle is to switch off the box. Studies have shown that watching TV not only fosters inactivity and sloth, it also encourages mindless and repetitive snacking, inspired by the drip-drip drumbeat of fast-food commercials. A University of Toronto nutritionist recently found that kids who watched TV while eating lunch consumed an extra 228 calories compared to those who ate without the television on. 'Eating while watching television overrides our ability to know when to stop eating,' reported the Canadian Institute for Health Research. In a similar study, the University of Michigan found that young children exposed to two or more hours of television a day were three times more likely to be overweight than kids watching for less than two hours.

Avoid Couch Potato Syndrome by keeping the TV in its place – in one room, not littered about the house on every available surface, as if you can't make it from the bathroom to the kitchen without finding out what's happening on *EastEnders*. Keep it mostly off. Turn it on when there's something specific to watch – look, I'm not Miss Jean Brodie and it doesn't have to be an edifying documentary about life in ancient Ur or how to install a composting loo. But it could be something useful or uplifting or funny or piquant. Something memorable. You can really slim down your TV times by deciding to stop watching – ooh, I don't know – *Property Fit Club*, about overweight people trying to do DIY. Stop watching *My Mother Was Built Like a Truck*, *Canine Masterchef*, *Honey, I Ate the Kids*, or whatever dross the box is spewing out this evening. Stop watching addictive telly – the sagas and soaps and series which sap your time and train you to need your nightly fix. Stop watching the eye-gouging pointlessness of reality TV shows, where you get to see basic life-forms pluck their eyebrows and argue about Cornflakes. Snub the TV talent shows that suck you in with the thrill of a phone vote for 65p. Don't watch the foxtrot. Learn it. It doesn't take a polymath to recognize that settling down for another evening of glazed gazing into one corner of the living room, illuminated by the spectral blue of the screen, is a waste of everything except energy.

TV also tends to present a fantasy world of perfection, where anyone can be famous just so long as they can fit into a very small dress – leaving the viewer feeling out of sorts and awfully susceptible to the pull of a cheering fatty snack. Oh, and if you do decide to watch TV, do it on an inflatable exercise ball. Do the same when you use your mobile. May as well tone while you phone.

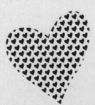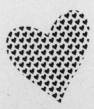

84 ALWAYS DO ONE MORE REP

The glory of exercise, no matter how piffling, is that in time you get fitter. Things that made you retch with exhaustion last month can feel like a breeze the next, as long as you stick with it. Don't think of it as a mountain to climb. It's not even a hill. It's more a slight incline. Before long, you'll be at the summit, looking down on the poor suckers below who didn't stir their sorry selves when you did. Here's how to start as you mean to go on:

✸**Exercise early**. It's the most effective strategy for keeping new recruits on track; people who work out in the morning are 40 per cent more likely to maintain the routine than those who postpone their workout until later in the day.

✸**Tell people**. That way you'll stick with it. While men tend to be goal-oriented, women are gossip-oriented. A team from the University of Hertfordshire tracked more than three thousand people attempting to achieve a range of things including weight loss. They found that women were more successful at keeping their resolutions if they told family and friends about their plans, thus increasing their chances of sticking with the programme by 10 per cent. Share, go public, and you've nowhere to hide.

✸**Incentivize**. This is one of my least liked words, second only to 'actioning' (though 'conversate' and 'deliverables' put up a pretty strong fight). But it does refer to a necessary requirement for the successful uptake and maintenance of regular exercise. You need to feel you are progressing. You need to be heading towards a goal, rather than trolling about in ever-decreasing circles until you lose the will to live. Incentives will help. Run to work for a month and spend the saved petrol money or travel fares on a new pair of twinkly shoes. Swim every day for a week and claim your lie-in at the weekend, leaving the family to find the fridge on their own. Actor Michelle Ryan relies on the encouragement of the *Rocky* soundtrack; for you, it might be Prodigy or Prokofiev at full blast. Alternatively, try a Garmin running monitor – a clever watch which relays your heart rate, speed, GPS position and route back to your laptop, so that you can compare today's effort with yesterday's. Go on. Be proud. It's a much underrated vice.

✳ **If motivation doesn't work, try coercion**. Put a contract on yourself at stickK.com. The website – dreamed up by an economics professor at Yale – acts as a 'commitment store' whereby you specify your aim and stake money on it. If you achieve the goal, the money comes back to you; if you fail, it goes to charity and you feel like a schmuck. Though it is largely dependent on self-regulation, you can add the frisson of peer pressure by opting to have progress emails sent to family and friends, allowing your sister in Geneva to know if you've been lingering too long at the dessert trolley. Professor Dean Karlan, co-founder of stickK, explains that the commitment-contract concept is based on two well-known principles of behavioural economics: 'One, people don't always do what they claim they want to do; and two, incentives get people to do things.'

'Run to work for a month and spend the saved petrol money or travel fares on a new pair of twinkly shoes.'

✳ **Look the part**. I have taken to walking the children to school wearing my mildly snazzy gym kit, all elastane and proper running shoes. This way, I arrive at the gates looking halfway decent, calm before the storm, and no one gets to see the 'after' picture, when my face has turned a curious ruby-red and sweat has puddled upon my upper lip. After a stiff run around the rec, I take the back route home and only ever meet one man and his dog. The dog casts pitying glances in my direction. But who cares? It's a dog.

✳ **Get real at the gym**. Of *course* everyone is looking at you. But they're also looking at everyone else. You may just hear tiny sighs of relief as people clock signs of cellulite, stretch marks, rampant bikini lines. The objective of the gym is to look great later, not at the time.

✴ **Learn to love your sweat**. Take a tip from men, who have long known that there is status in sweat. But it has to be in the right place. At the gym, the wrong places include anywhere too close to your exercising neighbour – sweat, like retsina, doesn't travel well – or on back rests and handrails.

✴ **Talk test yourself**. If you can comfortably hold a sustained conversation (or sing) during exercise, you're not working hard enough to gain aerobic benefit. Give your mouth a rest and work those glutes. If that all sounds too manic, relax. You really only need to . . .

85 KNOW THE POWER OF THE POTTER

Scientists at the University of Missouri-Columbia have found that 'pottering about' is just as valuable and effective an exercise as pounding away in the gym. Ha ha! The research team discovered that many of the physiological changes in the body that arise between total inactivity and 'pottering about' are more extreme than those between pottering and more strenuous exercise. What pleasant news. It may even call for mild celebration – a jig, perhaps, or a whoop. Or a nice cup of tea with my friend Alfred over at the allotments, a man whose body barometer is set permanently to Potter Mode, a pace he has found to be perfect for the cultivation of runner beans, dahlias and a general sense of bonhomie.

A further survey, this time of almost twenty thousand Scots, found that just twenty minutes of moderate exercise, such as gardening or housework, *once a week*, boosts one's mood – and daily physical activity is linked to lower stress levels all round. So let's hear it for pottering – the ideal way to dispel crushing metaphysical angst!

While puttering like an engine at traffic lights is beneficial in so many ways, sadly the same does not apply to sitting on your tush. The researchers found that lipase, an enzyme which helps the body break down fat, is suppressed, almost to the point of shutting off, after a day without movement. When people sit – in front of a TV, a monitor, a computer game, a fifteen-hour *Ring* cycle at La Scala – fat is more likely to be stored as adipose tissue than be passed to the muscles, where it can be burned. Sitting for prolonged periods thus results in the retention of fat, a lower HDL (that's the 'good cholesterol') and an overall reduction in the metabolic rate. Boo.

BURN BABY BURN:
CHART YOUR ENERGY EXPENDITURE

If you did sweet FA all day, lying in bed and dozing, your own body would naturally burn roughly 1,400 calories a day. This happens without you even noticing and is called the average base metabolic rate; it amounts to just under a calorie a minute for an average-sized woman (67 kg). Irritatingly enough, men burn more – around 1,700 a day (or 1.2 calories per minute) if they are of average size (81 kg). You can up the ante considerably by adding bursts of activity to your day. For instance:

Activity	Burn (in calories)
Sprint for the bus (one minute)	18
Browse shops for half an hour	68
Kiss in desultory fashion for ten minutes	11
Play air guitar to whole of Lynyrd Skynyrd's 'Free Bird'	250
Apply morning make-up for ten minutes	33
Run eight-minute miles for half an hour	350*
Have a 45-minute manicure	50
Push supermarket trolley for half an hour	83
Vacuum the living room. Properly. Under the sofa too	58
Play golf for half an hour	105
Do yoga for half an hour	91

Clubbing, intensive	257
Perform karaoke, for instance:	
The Carpenters' 'Yesterday Once More'	10.1
The Beatles' 'Let it Be'	11.4
Frank Sinatra's 'My Way'	15.6
Guns 'n' Roses' 'Sweet Child O' Mine'	21
Nintendo Wii, half an hour	75
Chew gum	11
Chew gum and fart at the same time	15.3
Fidget for a bit	10

All figures are approximate and are burned in excess of normal resting metabolism.

*The number of calories required to run a kilometre is, handily enough, equivalent to your weight in kilograms – so a runner of 71 kg will burn 71 calories/km. Isn't that neat? I also like the fact that your height is around three times the circumference of your head. And that your foot length is approximately the distance from your elbow to your wrist. Not strictly relevant, I grant you, but pleasing none the less.

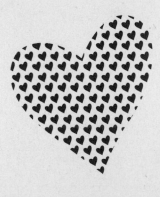
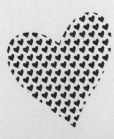

86 HAVE MORE ENERGETIC SEX

You probably think that everyone's at it. All the time. Banging away like Keith Moon. Coming like there's no tomorrow. Sex, more than any other human activity, is prey to Room B Syndrome – the feeling that there's a wild party going on next door and you're just not on the guest list. It's a fallacy, of course, promoted by unrealistic media chit-chat and bogus 'research' by companies who want to sell you innovative sex toys. But despair not. Recent figures show that on average British people make love a few times a month.

The truth is if we indulged rather more often, we'd certainly be a fitter, saucier bunch. Beyond that, sex is well known to be a salve, a salvation. It releases oxytocin, which begets intimacy and battles insomnia. It can improve self-esteem, combat stress and also boost immunity to disease, linked as it is to higher levels of a natural antibody, immunoglobin A, which protects against colds and other infections. (Not exactly racy, I know. But interesting.) A half-hour romp uses around 150–200 calories – about double the burn of golf, and easily twice the fun. If you effect the 'Italian chandelier' sexual position, you will apparently consume up to 912 calories an hour. *Mamma mia!*

Clearly, there's more than just fun and frolics at stake here: tune in to your sex drive and you'll look better. Look better and you'll want more. See? It's one big circle o' love.

YES! YES! YES!
HOW TO HAVE MORE SEX

✴ Before you love your partner, love yourself. You are gorgeous. Really. Chant this in the shower. Tell it to the mirror. And know that a woman who is embarrassed about the size of her backside is about as erotic as a cold flannel. Most men are grateful for all mercies, not just small ones.

✳ Get to know your cycle. The one in the hall. Apparently, twenty minutes on an exercise bike can heighten a woman's sexual response. Cycling, in particular, improves circulation, which is the very crux of sexual function.

✳ Don't turn to food to turn you on. Dwell instead upon this anonymous thought: 'Food has replaced sex in my life; now, I can't even get into my own pants.' Let that be a lesson.

✳ But do eat well. Aphrodisiacs are, on the whole, worthless, though mildly entertaining on a long winter's night. According to Cambridge nutritionist Dr Toni Steer, 'Oysters are dead in the water: we know of no scientific evidence showing that any particular nutrients enhance sexual function or libido.' Bah. The best way to coax your libido up a notch is to eat a nutritionally balanced diet. I know, it's hardly rip-your-shirt-off sexy, is it? By way of consolation, some foods *do* support the natural production of oestrogen, which could help put a tingle in your jingle. These include pomegranate, fennel and soya milk, of which more in Chapter Ten. Asparagus and avocados are high in vitamin E (considered to be a sex-hormone stimulant), while you may improve the blood flow to your poontang with the allicin in garlic (eat it, for God's sake, don't rub it on). If you really want to get it on more often, ditch the triple-fudge ice-cream (it makes a dreadful mess of the mattress) and serve sex in a bowl instead. Take:

> 1 fennel bulb, sliced thin
> 1 orange, shucked of peel and pith, juice squeezed
> 1 pomegranate. The excavated ruby seeds are really quite fetching
> A handful of young mint leaves for colour and bite
> Chopped almonds for crunch (the aroma is also said to be a switch-on)
> Accessorize with a flute of Louis Roederer Cristal (optional)

Eat, kiss, *frotter*.

87 GIVE UP YOUR CAR

Use a pool instead (try a website such as liftshare.org.uk or streetcar.co.uk). Go on, live life in the fast lane! If your car is just too vital a component of your everyday existence – and I do understand how tempting it can be, sitting there in the driveway all shiny and capable – at least think about giving it a brief sabbatical. Hide your car keys every second Wednesday in the month. Never drive less than a kilometre (unless you are moving wardrobes or elderly relatives). Spill a skinny latte on the front passenger seat (you won't want to drive again until the smell has been dealt with by an expensive valet. I have done this: it works).

Really, it's worth lessening your reliance on the car for so many reasons – economical, ecological, ethical – but while you're dithering about and anticipating rain, suck on this: a study of eleven thousand Atlanta residents reported a correlation between driving and weight gain. According to the findings, each additional hour spent in a car per day is associated with a 6 per cent increase in the likelihood of obesity. So give your life a handbrake turn: STOP if you are driving to the shop that you can see from your own front door, STOP if you are driving to the gym, STOP if you are driving to lull your baby to sleep. Start to think before you drive.

88 SET YOURSELF AN ACHIEVEMENT TASK

✳ Enter a sponsored swimming competition and make your friends promise money. You'll be too embarrassed to give up.

✳ Sign up for a half-marathon or the breast cancer 5 km. How about climbing Kilimanjaro or walking the entire South Coast Path? You think I'm joking? Don't go harrumph. Go for it.

✷ Do a volunteer holiday. No more lounging by the pool with Marian Keyes. You could be wrestling roos in the Outback, rehabilitating orang-utans in Sarawak, counting whales in the Outer Hebrides. It's all good, clean, energetic fun and comes with made-to-measure halo. Find out more at responsibletravel.com, ecoteer.com, originalvolunteer.co.uk, peopleandplaces.com, yoursafeplanet.co.uk.

✷ Build something. A sailing boat. A brick-and-flint granary. A tree-house. A life-sized sculpture of Gary Lineker using cheese-and-onion crisps. A den for the kids. A bookshelf. A ha-ha. Make it something permanent, something that fills you with a righteous sense of pride. Try not to build Ikea furniture, which is impermanent and will fill you with a hideous sense of existential regret.

✷ Enter a competition for which you are ill-equipped. Break-dancing, perhaps, or kung-fu. Aim to be a black belt by Christmas.

FITNESS: NOT JUST IN THE MUSCLES, BUT IN THE MIND

Now, dear hearts, it's time to introduce you to one of my favourite pieces of research. It tops my list because it is pure and it is brilliant, and because it demonstrates a wildly provocative idea. The study, conducted by Harvard's psychology department, took eighty-four female hotel attendants from seven hotels, each of whom cleaned an average of fifteen rooms a day. They walked and pushed and knelt and scrubbed. They carried and lifted and tucked and polished. But 66 per cent of them reported not exercising regularly. More than 36 per cent said they got no exercise at all.

The researchers then divided the women into two groups, giving one set detailed information, in English and Spanish, about the calorie burn of activities such as vacuuming rugs and cleaning bidets. They even put up notices in communal areas explaining the excellent health benefits of such work. After a month, the tutored group perceived that they did more exercise than before, while the untutored group's responses were unchanged. Neither group had altered their actual level of activity.

But here's the spooky bit: despite no change in exercise level, the tutored group showed 'improvement on every single one of the objective health measures recorded: weight, body fat, body mass index, waist-to-hip ratio and blood pressure'. The women in the informed group had lost an average of two pounds, lowered their blood pressure by almost 10 per cent, and were significantly healthier than their uninformed sisters.

It appears, then, that mindset can influence metabolism. So tell me: what are you going to believe today?

89   LAUGH – IT USES UP ENERGY

There's plenty of evidence to support the claim that laughter is good for you. Apparently, as we chortle, muscles in the face and body stretch, blood pressure and pulse rise and fall, and we breathe faster which transports more life-enhancing oxygen through the body. Research shows that laughter also strengthens the immune system, reduces food cravings (woo hoo!) and increases your threshold for pain. A real honking belly laugh burns calories, tightens up the abs, diaphragm and shoulders, and, according to research presented at 2008's annual meeting of the American Physiological Society, reduces the amount of unruly cortisol coursing around your body. A simple smile exercises sixteen muscles in your face and increases the production of endorphins. Even a false smile can lift your mood. Try it.

Smiling more, looking on the bright side, walking on the sunny side – these will all help on a day beset by the blues. Find an exercise that makes you giggle. Badminton. Roller-disco. Play Twister. Heckle a stand-up. Do Powerplate (that vibrating machine which dispensed with four stone of Charlotte Church's baby weight, and which makes you laugh as soon as you climb on board). If it feels good, you'll do it more often.

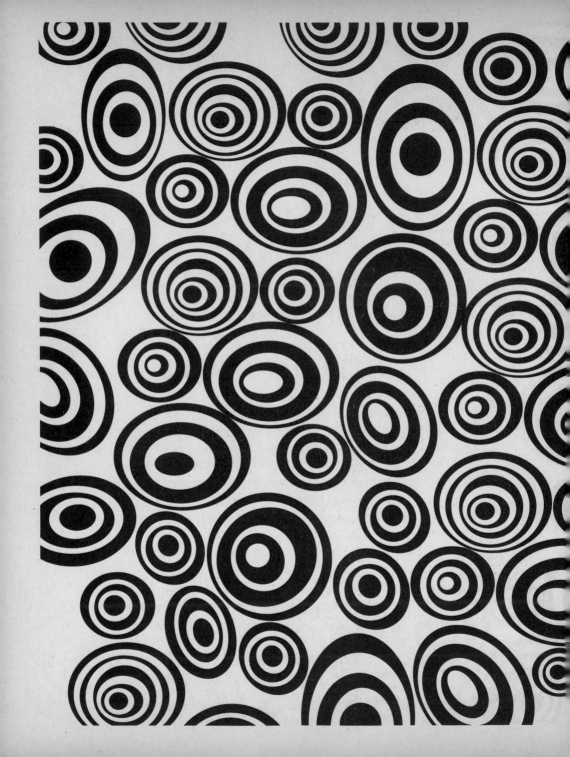

CHAPTER TEN
LIFE, THE UNIVERSE AND EVERYTHING
How All That You Do Reflects in the Mirror

Your body, your diet, your health – none of these fascinating things exists in a vacuum. Now that you're within sight of the finishing line, it's time to see that how you look, and, importantly, how you're perceived, is a function of a whole host of factors, some nebulous, some concrete. Your attitude. Your self-esteem. Your hormones. Your surroundings. Your agenda. All of this will dictate the shape you're in and how it feels to be there. Here's how to maximize your slim-line potential by harnessing all the lifestyle quirks, the ways of living, that will turn your body around and deliver a great new you.

90 KEEP YOUR HORMONES HAPPY

As Tammy so rightly said, sometimes it's hard to be a woman. What she didn't say, though it would have been helpful, is that most of our problems aren't to do with men. They're to do with hormones (I do appreciate that it wouldn't have made much of a song). You may not often dwell upon these ephemeral little doodads, but somewhere, everywhere, in the depths of your being, they control your metabolism, your destiny, your life; released by glands in the body, they have a multitude of overlapping, interweaving, fascinating functions, controlling all metabolic activities and basically calling the shots. We needn't go into the role of every blessed hormone here; what matters to us is that they affect calorie intake, nutrient uptake and energy expenditure – the three factors that dictate the body shape you inhabit.

Countless studies have examined the role of hormones in weight loss and gain. Insulin, cortisol, adrenalin, oestrogen, progesterone, DHEA – they all have an impact and it is in your best interests to find balance within to look better without. Losing fat is, after all, a biochemical process. It doesn't happen on the treadmill or at the fridge door. It happens in your cells.

Women are far more prone to fluctuating hormone levels than men, so it really pays to keep your hormones happy by eating hormone-enhancing and balancing foods which will give you a better chance of staving off fat deposition. According to Daniel Sister, a noted London doctor who specializes in hormone therapy, they will 'help satisfy hunger, reduce cravings, stimulate the release of fat-burning hormones, improve the efficiency of your digestion, increase energy levels . . .' They may even walk the dog if you ask them nicely. The idea is to reject inferior fuel and start putting premium-grade gas in your tank. So:

✱ Up your intake of vegetables, especially the cruciferous brassicas – kale, greens, broccoli, cabbage, cauliflower, pak choi, kohlrabi – all of which are particularly beneficial to your hormonal health. See below for how to cope with kohlrabi.

✳ Soya beans will be similarly beneficial. Use soya milk instead of cow's on your morning muesli; drink miso soup as an instant warmer; choose tofu as protein once a week (more if it appeals; if tofu seems bland, choose the firm variety and marinate it in soy sauce, chilli oil, ginger, garlic and chopped shallot; or try the tangier smoked version).

✳ Sesame seeds, though small, are full of hormone-harmonizing goodness. Falafel with hummus, tahini and shredded cabbage makes an excellent supper.

✳ Introduce more phyto-oestrogens (plant sources of oestrogen) into your diet – such as sprouted alfalfa, chickpeas, cherries, parsley, liquorice, linseed, rye, buckwheat, fenugreek, Korean ginseng. If this is all too complicated, simply turn to legumes, wholegrains, root vegetables, seeds and pulses. Or choose lentil soup (you've been doing this since Chapter Two, so you're already ahead of the curve).

✳ Avoid synthetic oestrogens (used to fatten cattle and increase egg and milk production) by choosing organic. Your aim is for hormonal balance, so try to eliminate 'oestrogenic' substances from your environment. These pollutants, which can be found in plastics, hair dyes and cosmetics among other things, are capable of mimicking the effects of oestrogen in the body. The symptoms of oestrogen dominance include water retention, breast tenderness, PMS, mood swings, depression, loss of libido, heavy or irregular periods, fibroids, cravings for sweets and – you guessed it – weight gain.

✳ In fact, renounce PMS and all its evil, self-loathing works; tablets of vitamin B-complex and capsules of evening primrose oil should help see it off. You could follow the example of Gwyneth Paltrow, who was advised to take brewer's yeast and eat more wholegrains to get added vitamin B6 into her diet.

✳ Include more essential fatty acids in your diet. So, more oily fish – mackerel, tuna, sardines, herring and salmon – sticking within recommended weekly guidelines. This is particularly important for women who have PMS because the gamma linoleic acid in omega oils can help iron out hormonal mood swings, leaving your vases and your marriage intact. If you're a vegetarian, get added EFAs from flax- or hemp-seed oil.

✳ Zinc-rich foods are hormone helpers. You'll find zinc in red meat, liver, nuts, dried fruit and oysters.

✳ Exercise not only tones the body, raises muscle mass, releases anxiety and maintains cardiovascular health and bone density, it also affects the hormone systems in the body, by, among other things, increasing the responsiveness of cells to insulin and helping to metabolize cortisol and adrenalin, turning your body from one that stores fat into one that burns it. Retrieve those trainers and make a start today.

'The American Association of Indexers, based in Albuquerque, New Mexico, has taken kohlrabi as a mascot, because 'no one knows who we are, or what to do with us either'.

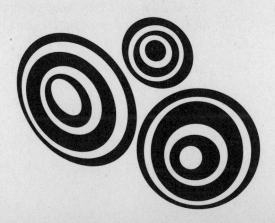

COPING WITH **KOHLRABI**

Kohlrabi, I discovered just recently, is enormously good for you – stuffed with hormone-loving compounds, cancer-fighting phytochemicals, masses of potassium and good old-fashioned vitamin C. But what exactly is it? And once you know what it is, what exactly do you do with it?

It turns out that the 'kohlrabi question' is widespread. No one can quite work out its purpose; it is the Prince Edward of the vegetable world. Even Nigel Slater, the king of the kitchen, is left floundering: 'I am honestly not sure what to say to those of you who have emailed, somewhat hopefully, about what to do with this particular veg,' he writes. 'At the risk of asking for trouble from the kohlrabi fan club, I must admit this one defeats me.'

Curiously, there *is* a kohlrabi fan club. The American Association of Indexers, based in Albuquerque, New Mexico, has taken this modest vegetable as a mascot, because 'no one knows who we are, or what to do with us either'.

Kohlrabi, then, is not the new Iranian president. It is not a Samurai torture technique. It is a vegetable, most commonly used as cattle feed. Yum. According to its apologists, kohlrabi has 'delicious leaves that are tender and excellent in salads or stir-fried'. The bulb is 'naturally sweet and can be eaten raw or steamed or shredded into soups and salads'. It is also a welcome addition to the cheese board, to be eaten raw, like an apple. I should warn you that it tastes mildly of drains. But then so do truffles, and it never did them any harm.

FAT AT FORTY:
YOUR BODY'S HORMONAL WEIGHT-BOMB

As Nora Ephron rightly warns in her book *I Feel Bad About My Neck*: 'At the age of fifty-five, you will get a saggy roll just above your waist even if you are painfully thin. This saggy roll will be especially visible from the back and will force you to re-evaluate half the clothes in your closet, especially the white shirts.' This, alas, is something that happens to us all. It's even happening to Elizabeth Hurley. 'The biggest change at forty is that you can't stay slim with yoga or Pilates alone,' she confessed recently. 'You have to do something aerobic unless you don't eat much. But I eat lots.'

When professional hard-bodies like Hurley are experiencing the treacle-slow-down of life, you know something's up. As one wag put it, 'The older you get, the tougher it is to lose weight, because by then your body and your fat are *really good friends*.'

The bitter truth is that everything flags in middle life. Says hormone doctor Daniel Sister, 'The first few pounds may mysteriously appear when you hit your mid-thirties – regardless of how much you eat or how much you exercise. Muscle tissue decreases and your body's basal metabolic rate begins to slow down. Your ability to burn calories is reduced, like a poorly burning chimney. A few years ago, research finally validated what we long ago suspected: fat cells have a gender. A woman's fat cells are physiologically different from a man's. They are larger, more active and more resistant to dieting. As women enter their middle years, in response to lower oestrogen levels, their 30–40 billion fat cells increase in size, number and ability to store fat.' The upshot, and crushing downside, of all this is that menopausal women are highly efficient fat storers – and the belly is usually where everything goes to pot. All the more reason, then, to get in touch with your hormones and treat them with respect.

91 AIM FOR LESS STRESS

Here's a surprise: our demanding, challenging, competitive lifestyles have an enormous impact on our weight and shape. Rushed, stuffed eating, unpredictable mealtimes, low-grade nutrition – all of this has its pernicious effect, as evidenced in a study of sixty women at Yale University. Researchers found that abdominal fat develops when a person is under long-term stress, thanks to the release of cortisol. This hormone is produced during a fight-or-flight response, stimulating insulin release and promoting rapid fat and carb metabolism to cope with extreme demands. This serves to increase your appetite for high-starch, high-fat foods. So, if you are under constant stress – and nearly one in ten of us report that we are experiencing work-related stress to the extent that it is making us ill – cortisol levels are persistently elevated and, lo and behold, you always fancy a fry-up.

'There's good evidence to suggest that cortisol activates an enzyme which promotes fat storage in fat cells (adipocytes),' explains Dr Joanne Lunn, nutrition scientist at the British Nutrition Foundation. 'The number of receptors for cortisol is greater in intra-abdominal adipocytes, so the accumulation of fat at this site will be accentuated when levels of cortisol are high.' In other words, stress turns women into apples. It also, adds Emma Stiles, nutritional scientist at the University of Westminster, 'increases insulin and decreases female hormones', with all the waist thickening we already know this entails.

In a related study, researchers at the University of California found that stressed-out rats responded by drinking increasingly more sugar water and eating increasingly more lard. They got fat by cushioning themselves with 'comfort' food. This, then, is why doughnuts always seem so consolatory, and why Homer Simpson has them as a primary food group. ('Stressed' backwards spells 'desserts', as Homer himself might say.)

Oh, and to top it all like whipped cream on a sundae, stress also depletes all manner of beneficial nutrients – from the antioxidant vitamins (A, E, C, and vitamin B-complex) to minerals such as zinc, selenium, calcium, magnesium, iron, potassium, sulphur and molybdenum. Without those? Honey, you'd be nothing.

The goal here, then, is to let go a little. If you march through life with gritted teeth, heart palpitations and a tense nervous headache, if you are certain that everything will fall apart if your pencils aren't lined up, it's time to engage in some stress management. Play squash, lift weights, meditate, spend time in a bubble bath and come up smelling of roses. If none of this helps, talk to a health professional.

92 SLEEP WELL

Are you sitting comfortably? Then, let me introduce you to Leptin and Ghrelin. They may sound like characters from Rivendell or the Shires, but these two are hormones, and here's what they do.

✷ **Leptin** is the way your fat speaks to your brain. And what a profoundly fascinating conversation that must be. Leptin's role is to keep the hypothalamus informed about the adequacy of your energy stores; it's the satiety hormone. If the signal falters, the brain seeks a source of energy to fill the void. It boosts hunger and sends you off on a hunt for that chicken drumstick in the fridge. To make matters worse, a large fat cell, being large, produces a lot of leptin. When we diet, those fat cells shrink (the accumulated effect is what you marvel at in the mirror), and leptin levels fall. In a galling negative feedback, this stimulates your hunger and encourages your body to conserve energy. Arrrgh.

✷ **Ghrelin**, as we already know, is produced in the stomach to signal hunger to the brain, a hormonal version of a tummy rumble.

What, you may wonder, has all this to do with sleep? Well, leptin has a circadian rhythm and reaches its peak during sleep. If you're not sleeping well (and around a third of us don't), peak leptin levels are not reached and the brain sends out its foot soldiers – hunger pangs and energy conservation – just as it does when your fat cells shrink during dieting. At the same time, lack of sleep causes ghrelin levels to rise. Your appetite gets a hike and the cookie jar calls.

There have been innumerable – sometimes controversial, sometimes hyperbolic – investigations into the effects of leptin and ghrelin on weight. A précis might include:

✳ Stanford's study of a thousand volunteers, which found that those who slept fewer than eight hours a night had lower levels of leptin and higher levels of ghrelin, and (here's the rub) they also had higher levels of body fat. 'Specifically, those who slept the fewest hours per night weighed the most.'

✳ A study at the University of Warwick found that sleep deprivation was associated with almost double the risk of being obese.

✳ Researchers at Bristol University compared blood samples from insomniacs and good sleepers. The former had leptin levels 15 per cent below, and ghrelin levels 15 per cent above, normal.

✳ A study at Laval University in Quebec found that there may be an ideal sleep zone of around eight hours a night that facilitates body-weight regulation.

✳ Professor Jim Horne, of Loughborough University's renowned Sleep Research Centre, counsels caution in all of this, noting 'It seems that, at best, sleep plays a minor physiological role in causing obesity, although there may be a more behavioural explanation, for example, via sleeplessness-induced lassitude and "comfort eating".'

Either way, what you need to absorb is that sleep is not just a passive zombie state; it is active, intricate and vital to the smooth running of your metabolism. If we disrupt it with a twenty-four-hour lifestyle, over-stimulating ourselves in the dead of night, working double shifts and long hours, eating at odd times, our bodies will inevitably suffer.

Whatever our hormones are up to, poor sleep will certainly rob us of the energy required to bounce out of bed and bite the day. This low-energy cycle is the arch-enemy of sustained weight loss, turning us on to sugar snacks and caffeine pick-ups to get us through ... which then serve to interrupt sleep patterns and so the whole sorry saga goes on and on.

By now you should be feeling pretty sleepy. Great. Go to bed. Sweet dreams. Not too sweet, mind.

HOW TO **SLEEP EASY** IN YOUR BED

According to the Sleep Council, two-thirds of people believe that they get less sleep now than they did a few years ago – around 90 minutes less, according to one leading US sleep expert. 'You probably have a generation that is quite sleep disturbed,' agrees Kathleen McGrath, medical director of Sleep Matters, a helpline operated by the Medical Advisory Service. 'I think we are looking at a time bomb. People now are not physically tired but mentally tired ... Some people's bedrooms look like the Starship *Enterprise*, lit up with TV screens and computers. Your bedroom is for two things: for sleep and for sex, not necessarily in that order.'

If you toss and turn and clock-watch, your body is not getting the rest it so richly deserves. Professor Jim Horne has the following tips for restful sleep:

✱ **Pack up your troubles**. Anxiety and over-stimulation will interfere with sleep, so do soporific, absorbing tasks before bed. Not TV, which is a stimulant. Reading is the classic method. Horne also recommends jigsaws, walking the dog, knitting and washing up. Your kitchen will sparkle, and you might end up with a nice new scarf.

✱ **Rise at a regular time**. No matter when you went to sleep, get up at the same time each day. This helps to programme your body clock into a good sleep-wake pattern which, says Professor Horne, can be hugely helpful for insomniacs.

You don't need forty winks. Try fifteen. If you're feeling shattered by mid-afternoon, take only a short fifteen-minute nap. Beyond that, you'll eat into your body's sleep needs and disrupt your night.

Keep it cool. Your body needs to cool down during sleep. So no mega-tog duvets, electric blankets, fuggy central heating. Nudge open the window.

Go sssh. Heavy curtains, eye masks, ear plugs, blackout blinds – do what it takes to navigate light and noise pollution. If your BlackBerry sleeps beside you, put it outside. Leave laptops off and banish them downstairs.

Clock off. Melatonin can help reset the body clock, according to Dr Daniel Sister. It's a hormone produced in the pineal gland to regulate sleep and wake cycles, but can be taken as a supplement (available over the counter in the States, but only on prescription or online in Europe) to help promote lovely lullaby sleep.

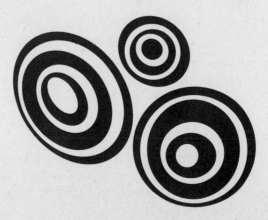

STOP THINKING BIG AND TALKING BALONEY

Never utter phrases such as:

✳ '**I've got a sweet tooth**.' No, you are addicted to sugar. A note to all sucrophiles out there: science has recently decreed that there is no such thing as a sweet tooth. Researchers at Duke University in North Carolina claim that the human brain 'senses' that sweet foods are high in calories and 'rewards' people when they eat them by releasing hormones that make them feel happier. It's not your tooth, sweetie, it's your brain. Train your brain, junk the junk.

✳ '**I've got a big appetite**.' Perhaps you have. But that's a confession, not an excuse.

✳ '**I have a slow metabolism**.' So move about more to burn more calories.

✳ '**I am absolutely ravenous . . . I could eat my own liver! I am starving . . . my blood sugar is dangerously low . . . If I don't eat that cherry bakewell right now, I'm going to pass out!**' No you're not. I'm guessing it's mere moments since your last meal. Get a hold of yourself, woman. If you find that your blood sugar suffers mad spikes and troughs, even it out by eating low-glycaemic-index foods such as nuts or prunes or stoneground wholemeal toast, not refined carbohydrates like cakes or cookies. These will simply add to the rollercoaster ride and send you over the edge in a hail of pie crumbs.

✳ '**Woo hoo! Broken biscuits! That means all the calories have leaked out!**' This aphorism, and others like it, is not even faintly amusing. It is what greedy people say to cross the bridge between one Ginger Nut and the next.

✳ '**I would rather be big and happy than on a diet and miserable**.' I like the second clause of this sentence, but *big and happy*? More like fat and delusional. Don't diet, but *do* be honest with yourself.

✻ '**I have big bones**.' Yup. And so does a woolly mammoth. What's your point?

✻ '**I was born fat**.' Good grief. Where to start?

✻ '**It's just middle-age spread**.' Trust me, that's the worst kind.

✻ '**I'm eating for two now**.' If you are pregnant, all the more reason to stay healthy. Don't reach for the chocolate mini-rolls as soon as the stick turns blue. You'll regret it all in about . . . ooh, forty weeks' time.

✻ Stop starting sentences with '**I always** . . .' Surprise yourself. I always do.

94 GET INTO THE GOOD LIFE AND GROW YOUR OWN VEGETABLES

Why? I'll give you ten good reasons:

✻ **Taste**. Home-grown carrots. Try them. You'll see. You'll eat more. You'll see.

✻ **Thrift**. Why pay three pounds for a bag of rocket when you can grow masses of it on the patio for pennies?

✻ **Control**. You're in charge of what you spray on your lettuces. There's no multinational conglomerate breathing fumes all over them and shovelling on pesticide and then keeping them in a lock-up for months on end before they even meet a mouth. They are yours, all yours! Thus, unlike many a bag of shop-bought, chlorine-washed salad, they're packed with weight-erasing vit-C vitality.

✻ **Jamie Oliver**. He does it, so you can too.

✱ Eco-cred. No packaging. No food miles. No guilt. Get into composting and you're more ethical still. I would recommend a wormery, but, really, *euuch*. In the *house*? I prefer to chuck organic waste into a hot composter, which manages to chow its way through egg-shells, tea-bags, chicken bones, all sorts – though not through silver teaspoons from the set you were given as a wedding present by Aunt Evelyn. That was a relief, I can tell you.

✱ Chill. This is slow food – which, as we know already, makes it good food. It is necessarily local and seasonal. And it's relatively easy . . . so long as you remember to water your pumpkins, thin out your lollo rosso, pinch out runner beans, prick out seedlings, earth up potatoes. OK, so you may need a book. I recommend Carol Klein's *Grow Your Own Veg* (BBC Books).

✱ Exercise. Weed the garden for half an hour and you'll motor through 150 calories. You'll probably need a manicure afterwards (that's fifty more).

✱ Wellies. Yes, the foundation of many a lovely outfit – particularly when paired with a rustic linen apron, a floral-sprigged dress, forget-me-nots entwined in your hair, that kind of thing. I'm all for trugs and clogs and homemade lemonade served in the garden on a warm day, perhaps with mismatched china and Aunt Evelyn's teaspoons. It's so quintessentially English, so Vita Sackville-West, so 'honey still for tea'. Get this growing lark right and you'll look as though you've strolled nonchalantly from the pages of *World of Interiors*, clutching a dibber and smelling of rhubarb compote. Such joy, and a fashion triumph to boot.

✱ Camaraderie. If you have never announced your arrival at a friend's house with a bag of home-grown leeks, you've never lived. These days, you may well find that an endless parade of acquaintances bring boxes of fruit and veg and homemade sloe gin to your door; Britain is now thought to be growing as much at home as it did during the Second World War, when lawns were dug up and people kept chickens in window boxes. This is a weight-loss dream – far better than arriving with a box of Cadbury's Roses.

✳ **Boasting rights**. If you have an allotment, you are a lucky minx indeed – forget an Hermès Birkin; what the *beau monde* really crave right now is a patch of tilled land upon which to sow perpetual spinach and curly kale. Though there are roughly 330,000 allotment-holders in the UK, as many as 100,000 are on allotment waiting lists at any one time. Feel free to use your hoe to fight off the competition, knowing your body is reaping the benefit.

95 BECOME A BUDDHIST AND END DESIRE. OR FOLLOW THE TAO AND DO NOTHING

Now that we're nearing our destination on this journey to figure-happy bliss, it's worth asking yourself some philosophical questions. Do you always want more? Are you never satisfied? Are you sad and hungry? I only ask because these aching, yearning sentiments have come to typify life in the twenty-first century. I'm not about to get all 'Confucius, he say' on your ass. But there is a lesson to be learned from the chronicles of ancient wisdom which will affect your relationship with everything in your world, including your lunch. The crux is to live consciously. With awareness. I know I sound like a fortune cookie, but this is important. It has to do with grand old chestnuts such as self-acceptance, responsibility and purposeful living. If you have already switched off and switched on the TV, just pause it. For a moment. Could you be kinder to yourself? Could you like yourself a little more? Could you tune in to something a bit more constructive than the notch on your belt?

In truth, we all could. There's no need to get fanatical about this, mind. According to idle rumour, Gwyneth Paltrow has in the past tried dining quite naked while sitting in the lotus position in front of a mirror, in order to facilitate an increase in self-awareness. You may find this somewhat trying if you have guests over for supper. Better, perhaps, to concentrate on something more meaningful than your own belly button. As Cyril Connolly wrote in *The Unquiet Grave*, 'The one way to get thin is to re-establish a purpose in life.' And, had he thought about it, I'm sure he would have added that the purpose ought *not* to be to 'have better buttocks' or 'get into a smaller bikini'.

When you stop to think – and I urge you to, right now – most of us could do with connecting more and criticizing ourselves less. In this respect, I'm with Henry Miller who said that 'the aim of life is to live, and to live means to be aware, joyously, drunkenly, serenely, divinely aware'.

We could, if we chose, live more in the present tense, here and now, not there and next. Interestingly, Buddha had plenty to say on the subject of body shape. 'What we think we become' was one of his. And my own personal favourite when things are crap and the dress doesn't fit: 'You can search throughout the entire universe for someone who is more deserving of your love and affection than you are yourself, and that person is not to be found anywhere. You yourself, as much as anybody in the entire universe, deserve your love and affection.'

PUT A LITTLE LOVE ON YOUR FORK

Food really ought to be served with soul, love and laughter, not peppered with caution, misgivings and guilt. There's so much enjoyment in a shared hot pot, a celebration cake, an innocent bowl of jelly and ice-cream . . . really, thinking about it all too hard, weighing it up and worrying about the consequences, simply sours the taste. Wouldn't it be better to rejoice?

By way of example, singing and eating always went hand in hand in our house when I was growing up (although it was well known that the pairing was considered rude in polite company). Still, when sausages were popping in the pan, or a roast chicken was sitting on its roost waiting to be carved, all manner of singing would break out. *Nessun Dorma*. The aria from Delibes's *Lakmé*. 'My Old Man Said Follow The Van'.

But, mostly, we sang when doing the washing-up, a nod to the well-known fact that singing makes a dull job go faster. My sister and I would do Abba, or hits from the musicals, with my mother doing her impromptu rendition of Nancy in *Oliver!*, all oom-pah-pah and Mr Percy Snodgrass, while she wiped down the Formica. My father preferred snippets of opera sung to his own libretto ('Toreador, don't spit upon the floor! Use the spittoon, that's what it's for!' addressed to the sticky chicken glue from the roasting pan). At Christmas, carols echoed around the steaming kitchen as the aunts and cousins, each clutching a damp tea towel, belted out 'Good King Wenceslas' or 'We Three Kings' and pirouetted across the lino in an attempt to avoid wiping up the heavy saucepans.

It was during one of these family get-togethers that I had a teenage wobble about what to wear out that evening to a disco (yes, it was that long ago). My grandmother, a woman well versed in the value of golden dancing shoes, said in her no-nonsense way, 'I wouldn't worry, darling, nobody's going to be looking at you.'

It has taken me years to realize that she meant it not unkindly, but as a call for me to be less *involved* with myself. Since then, I've discovered scientific studies which show that my grandmother was dead right: people aren't paying half as much attention to you as you think they are. Most of the time, they're bound up in an infinitely more fascinating subject. Themselves. So here's the thing. Sing more. Worry less. Remember that the person on the dance floor who looks as though she's having the best time, probably is.

96 FIGURE OUT THAT FRIENDS CAN BE FAT MAGNETS

Just last week, I spent a lunch-hour (more like three hours, but why quibble?) with friends Pippa and Lou. We were in high spirits, and all felt rather hedonistic and conspiratorial as we dipped great chunks of salty focaccia into a central pool of olive oil. We all decided to have starters because, well, weren't we celebrating something? No? Oh well, why not?

Three large glasses of Chilean Sauvignon Blanc later, Pip had ordered risotto, Lou had the confit de canard, so – what the hell? – I ordered the linguine carbonara. I thought a side of fat chips would be opportune, just to share. It would barely be six chips each. We ordered pudding because no one was watching, and then we ate the chocolate mints which accompanied coffee, because . . . well, who could remember why? There might have been a second bottle of white. And suddenly, what do you know? We were *shopping* . . .

Ah, bless 'em. It's not that girlfriends mean to make you eat and shop with such cavalier abandon. It's just that *you* doing it condones *them* doing it, which means *you* do it, and so the happy, fatty carousel goes round and round until you end up in a gigglesome heap on the floor.

Brian Wansink, in one of his many brilliant experiments, discovered recently that an especially good way to gain weight is to dine with other people. In *Mindless Eating – Why We Eat More Than We Think*, he reports that 'on average, those who eat with one other person eat about 35 per cent more than they do when they are alone; members of a group of four eat about 75 per cent more; those in groups of seven or more eat 96 per cent more . . . If you want to lose lots of weight, look for a thin colleague to go to lunch with (and don't finish the food on her plate).'

In fact, it can work both ways, particularly among women. As a rule, we tend to calibrate our restaurant order quite finely with what other women at the table have chosen, the gluttony or abstinence of the occasion being precisely socially sanctioned.

In my experience, and to corroborate Wansink's research, if the first bid is fairly high (a risotto primavera, say), the players will indeed go on to trump each other, adding side orders of buttered new potatoes and extra portions of hand-cut chips, until the final one to go finds herself in the embarrassing position of having ordered the entire left-hand side of the menu.

And yet, the whole game can play out differently. In what might be called the Beckhamist Twist, if Philippa kicks off with 'just a *tricolore*', Jodie will have the same, but with the dressing *on the side*. Look upon it as a sort of gastronomic gazundering. It all depends on the friends (underbidding is very popular in fashion circles) and the opening bid. Working logically, if six fashion editors go out for lunch, the last one to order could well go home hungry, possibly resorting to stealing the Mint Imperials from the bowl at the door to sustain her through till tea (yes, that was me).

The more at ease you are, though, the more likely you are to indulge in piggery (which is why many of us gorge when eating alone). It's also why holidaying with friends is as dangerous as it gets, the shark-infested waters of your social map. I recently went away on a self-catering holiday with friends and the sheer quantity of food that was bought, discussed, consumed and discussed again was phenomenal. Every third minute, someone seemed to be nudging another spoonful of mashed potato on to my plate. We'd eat and pick and chat and then eat some more, the constant ongoing conversation being about what we were going to have for the next meal and how many Tunnock's Caramel Wafer bars were still left in the larder.

It's understandable, of course. Humans are social beasts. Feeding brings us together. Food is brilliantly celebratory and cohesive, a lip-smacking, heart-warming social glue. You can well imagine that in those long-ago caves, our ancestors sat around arguing about the relative merits of wild hog over raw bison for tea – and not worrying a jot if they looked a bit lardy in a loin-cloth. These days, though, if you are serious about keeping your figure under control, you need to find ways to be with friends without putting on a pot of weight – and without coming across as a supercilious bore who knows the calorie content of the table napkins. One good way to do it is to buy all your girlfriends this book. Then you'll be on the same page, so to speak.

BEWARE THE DIET BUDDY,
FOR SHE MEANS YOU NO GOOD

Diet buddies aren't always the faithful friends you need when you want to slim down. As one writer puts it, somewhat bleakly, losing weight is 'like entering a war zone. There are no more friends. Keep in mind that no one really wants you to succeed.' Personally, being of a more optimistic hue, I'd like to think that women have more solidarity than that – but, even so, it's worth keeping your wits about you when you hear any of the following:

✳ 'But I don't want to drink alone.'

✳ 'You don't need to lose weight!'

✳ 'I cooked it especially for you because I know how much you like treacle sponge with cream *and* custard.'

✳ 'Oooh, stay and finish the bottle.'

✳ 'I know you said you wanted a single scoop, but they were doing a brilliant offer on this triple-boule super-blow-out with extra toffee sauce, chopped nuts and those dear little mini marshmallows.'

✳ 'Have this last pancake, it's only going in the bin.'

You need to know that these are all the ploys of the saboteur. Tell her to back off or you'll start bringing your own grape-seed extract to supper. Beware, too, anyone who gorges on people gaining weight. More crucial, though, than avoiding the naysayers and the feeders is to do as you would be done by. As Balzac stated, 'The more one judges, the less one loves.' So stop appraising, stop weighing up your peers, stop competing, stop feeding your friends banoffee pie in the hope that they'll burst free from their annoyingly flimsy little camisole tops. And start with a modicum of kindness, remembering that what goes around . . .

WHY FAT FRIENDS ARE FATTENING

A study at the University of California recently showed that obesity spreads within social networks and that people with fat friends are 50 per cent more likely to be overweight than those who hang out with skinny people. Further research by economists at the University of Warwick, Dartmouth College and the University of Leuven found that people are powerfully but subconsciously influenced by the weight of those around them. It turns out that fattitudes are catching. It's all relative. If your friends and family regularly tuck into a bucket of deep-fried chicken wings, you'll inevitably do the same. If they go for the hyper-Slurpee at the movies, your mega-Slurpee starts to look paltry by comparison. Says Professor Andrew Oswald at Warwick, 'Rising obesity needs to be thought of as a sociological phenomenon not a physiological one. People are influenced by relative comparisons, and norms have changed and are still changing.'

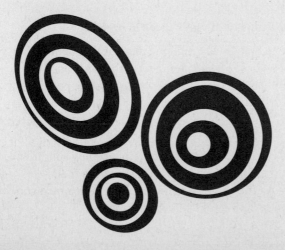

97 CHOOSE A CHALLENGE; DON'T GET TOO COSY

OK, you can't move continent or get engaged or divorced every time you feel your waistband get a bit tighter – but there is good evidence to suggest a seismic shift to your lifestyle is what will really change your shape. Don't get contented, like a milch cow. Don't settle, don't succumb, don't submit or slouch your way into an easy, acquiescent life.

'There is,' said Iris Murdoch, 'no substitute for the comfort supplied by the utterly-taken-for-granted relationship.' And a glorious thing it is too. But one of the greatest obstacles to weight-loss intentions is very often your partner, particularly if you have been in the relationship long enough to get thoroughly comfy, like a pair of old socks. If you're happy to burp in front of him, if you shave your legs while he shaves his chin, if you wash his boxers, then you are comfy (if you iron them, you're barking). But comfy is like a settee: squashy, stationary and quite hard to get out of.

Studies regularly show that women put on weight after they get married – partly because the prospect of that strapless organdie gown with cathedral train and matching bridesmaids is no longer blocking the view every time they look a cupcake in the face. But also because, once hitched, you tend to settle down, tuck in and order an extra portion of garlic bread. To coin an old proverb, as far as your figure is concerned, the most dangerous food is wedding cake. ('Matrimony,' said one astute observer, 'is a process by which a grocer acquires an account the florist had.')

Once married, it's all too easy to start eating big. Where once you'd have subsisted on a quick bowl of Alpen for supper, now you're cooking lamb chops and all the trimmings. You didn't used to *do* trimmings. Now you're making gravy! So why not spread the word? As the *Observer Food Monthly* magazine notes, 'Married people are feeders by nature. They do not fear carbohydrates, they get offended if you only eat half of everything . . . Beware the following: bread on side plates! Mash! Sauces! Married people love them.'

Once children are on the scene, your parental lifestyle (if that's not too grand a term for it) probably means that you stay in a bit more and go clubbing a bit less. House-bound, you're tied by some unseen umbilical cord to the biscuit tin and the bread basket. You sink the first glass of wine as soon as Olivia's little head hits the pillow, your reward for a day of motherly forbearance (and the fact that you managed to make an entire farmyard tableau from Play-Doh while putting three loads of washing on). Little wonder your pre-pregnancy jeans appear to have dropped in from another galaxy.

'If you're happy to burp in front of him, if you shave your legs while he shaves his chin, if you wash his boxers, then you are comfy.'

This isn't just idle observation. WeightWatchers recently produced a study of three thousand married women which revealed the different stages a female figure goes through over the course of a lifetime. Almost 66 per cent of those surveyed said their weight fluctuated depending on how happy they were at a specific time. According to the study, in the early days of a relationship, when a woman has found her dream man, she's 'so keen to impress that she even orders salad for a romantic meal'. Blimey. Next, she enters the Comfy Zone, when cosy nights in with her fella, a DVD and a Thai takeaway mean she'll pile on an average of 11.3 pounds. As the Big Day approaches, our heroine loses 9.2 pounds to squeeze into the Big Dress. The first baby brings many delights, among them an average 16 pounds of additional weight. Then, eventually, comes the Reinvention, when a woman realizes there is more to life than track pants and daytime telly. She drops more than a stone, whoopee, just in time for the peri-menopause to sabotage her plans . . .

How, then, to arrest the life-cycle lard? Your mission is to keep challenging yourself, stay out of ruts, shake up your life. If you always eat a huge meal with your partner, book in for a suppertime yoga class and make lunch your main meal of the day. If you find yourself doing the same things three evenings in a row, run to the end of the road and back as a penance. If your kids keep you in at night, take up piano or French or (better still) kick-boxing. Get a teach-yourself DVD: it will do you a darn sight more good than watching the entire five-season series of *The Wire*. Finally, once more to our old friend Honoré de Balzac: 'Marriage,' he wrote, 'must constantly fight against a monster which devours everything: routine.'

98 TAKE YOUR PASSIONS OFF THE PLATE

If the thought that gets you most exercised in life is whether you'll fit into the new stock arriving in Harvey Nicks, then you need to recalibrate things a bit. Who knows where your energies could take you once you stop fretting and fussing about your own sweet self . . . Fund-raising? Mucking out the donkey sanctuary? Keeping bees? Overthrowing the state? It matters little what it is, but, with this wholesale overhaul of your life and behaviour (look, you're at Number Ninety-eight; there's no stopping you now), you should be in the market for refocusing your attentions away from the size of your rump and on to something that might make the world one speck better. If you're going to get intense, ardent, fervent, far better that the object of your attentions is something that really matters (your favourite charity, a local youth club, a fund-raiser for trees to be planted at the end of your street. Go on, plant the trees yourself). You'll be surprised how much your body will benefit from a viewpoint that looks out, not in.

DEATH AND CHOCOLATE:
HOW MORBID THOUGHTS BREED HUNGER PANGS

Sometimes, a piece of research comes along that allows you to stand back and marvel at the incomparable intricacy of the human condition. Here's just such a study: according to new research at Rotterdam's Erasmus University, people who are thinking about their own deaths have an urge to consume more.

A paper published in the *Journal of Consumer Research* reveals that 'consumers, especially those with a lower self-esteem, might be more susceptible to over-consumption when faced with images of death during the news or their favorite crime-scene investigation shows'. They explain this effect using a theory called 'escape from self-awareness'. When people are reminded of their inevitable mortality, they may start to feel uncomfortable about what they have achieved in their lives and whether they have made a significant mark on the universe. One way to deal with such an uncomfortable state is to escape from it, by having another generous handful of Jelly Bellies. The lesson here is to dwell not upon death, but on the life in you yet (I did actually get that one from a fortune cookie).

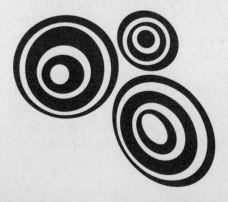

99 TAPE A PICTURE OF BAD BRITNEY TO YOUR FRIDGE

Britney's soulmate Madonna has this to say on the subject of body management: 'If you want to know how I look like I do, it's diet, exercise and being constantly careful.' Constantly. Careful. Clearly, most of us inhabit the intermediate territory, lodged in a halfway house somewhere between Bad Britney and Meticulous Madge. But we all need regular nudges and prompts to remind us of the game plan, recognizing that saying 'No!' to the pie has an immediate cost (no pie!) but – like flossing or pension plans – little immediate benefit. The benefit will come, with luck and a fair wind, tomorrow and tomorrow and tomorrow. To remind yourself of this, leave the wedding invitation on the mantelpiece, the cocktail dress hanging on the back of the bedroom door, the bikini shot taped to the tub of vanilla in the freezer. It's well worth keeping one eye on the calendar too; there's nothing like a pool party in July to put you off that second sausage. A series of social deadlines will stay your hand as it wanders off in search of superfluous sustenance.

The idea here is to know your foe and keep it at bay using a combination of vigilance and exquisite sangfroid.

100 IN EXTREMIS, KNIT

You don't only eat when you're hungry. Eating can be a response to stress, fatigue, loneliness, euphoria, grief ... In particular, though, we eat when we're bored. Research has shown that half of adults do exactly this, reaching for a bag of Percy Pigs or cheesy Quavers simply because they'll occupy another small slot in the endless loop of your existence. It's Eeyore's approach to thistles, a robotic, repetitive response to the featureless tract of time between here and there. It's why most of us eat a ton of crisps and chocolate on a long car journey, and why a tea break at work seems to make the day go faster (especially if accompanied by a Penguin biscuit). Food, though, is not the solution, it's the fuel. It's meant to take you somewhere, not leave you stranded on a bean bag wondering where the day has gone. If you find comfort and solace in the crinkle-cut of a McCoy's oven-baked crisp, you really need to get out more. Find another crutch.

BOREDOM EATING: DO SOMETHING MORE INTERESTING INSTEAD

✳ When a food craving strikes, Hollywood actresses are said to reach for their knitting needles rather than a giant bag of pretzels – Julia Roberts and Uma Thurman both do it, and you can't move backstage at fashion shows for crochet hooks and cable-stitch needles. You can charm yourself with the knowledge that knitting is incredibly cool, thanks to a recent resurgence among Hoxtonites, anarchists and guerrilla-knitting groups such as Cast Off and Knitta (a gang which 'tags' statues around the world with subversive bits of knitting). You could even join a knitting circle. The winter nights will fly by, and you'll end up with an interesting muffler rather than an empty bag of Kettle Chips and a hollow void in your soul. Have a look at knitty.com.

✳ Chew gum. To paraphrase Lyndon B. Johnson, 'Like Gerald Ford, you can't eat and chew gum at the same time.'

✳ Give yourself a manicure – it'll take care of your hands till lunchtime. The same goes for watercolours, scrap-booking, bassoon lessons. Make your own Christmas cards, stroke a cat, sew an enormous quilt from scraps of discarded clothes and then auction it for charity. I really don't mind what you do, as long as it's not mindless mastication.

CHAPTER ELEVEN
LOVE THYSELF
Big Yourself Up to Slim Yourself Down

Almost twenty years in the style business have drawn me to one clear conclusion. How you look has, in truth, very little to do with your weight. But it owes everything to your confidence. Think about the women you admire, the ones who've got it and know exactly what to do with it. I'll stake a bet – a pair of my very best Jimmy Choos – that they exude confidence, spirit, verve. Building your confidence will breed a healthier relationship with food, and a better relationship with your body. This is what you came for. This is what you've got – an intimate, intuitive awareness that you are wonderful. You don't need your bathroom scales to tell you this. You know it, deep down, beneath the slimming embrace of that sensational dress you're wearing.

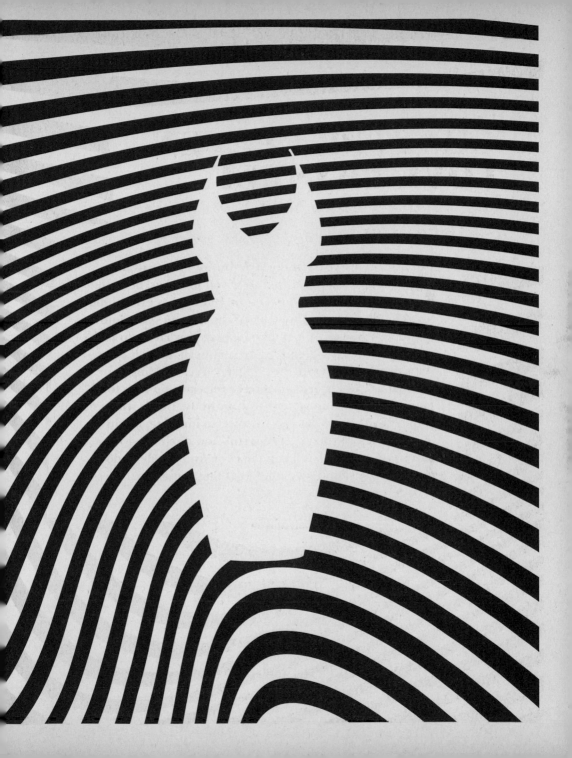

101 LOOK WITHIN TO TRIUMPH WITHOUT

Not long ago, I came across the word 'numinescence'. I have clasped it to my heart ever since and treasured it like the jewel that it is, despite the fact that somebody probably made it up – perhaps while watching the sun rise or drinking a third bottle of wine. A dictionary will tell you that the word 'numinous' can be applied to something that is 'awe-inspiring' or 'sublime', from the Latin 'numen' meaning deity. Numinescence, though, is more of a hybrid, a marriage of numen and luminescence. I like to think of it as '*it*', a quality intangible, timeless, transcendental, the thing that, if you could bottle it, would turn you into an instant billionaire.

Stick it in a bottle, though, and the whole lot would spoil. Being volatile and personal, it can't be bagged, labelled and shipped around the globe to be shoved on a shelf in Selfridges or Saks, no matter who tries. Numinescence, then, is the butterfly that cannot be caught, the gossamer glow of mystery, nuance and energy. You don't buy it with a credit card; you buy it with confidence. Confidence and love.

Consider Botox, by way of example. Why do women who have injected their faces with botulism always look so sour, so desperate, ironed of all glory? My feeling is that it's because they're afraid to inhabit their own face. This collapse in confidence shows, even through the taut shine of their skin. By contrast, think of women who know and enjoy themselves. You don't encounter many, not in an age devoted to undermining our self-belief and selling us a dream ticket in a squeezy bottle. But when you do, when you're in the presence of numinescence, it is memorable and affecting, your whirring mind trying to place what it was about that woman – her perfume? her smile? – that made her stay with you long after she'd left the room.

There are, of course, famous women who have it in their very soul. Cate Blanchett. Erin O'Connor. Nigella Lawson. Tilda Swinton. Julianne Moore has it. Helen Mirren's got it. Elizabeth Taylor would have been lost without it. Catherine Zeta Jones appears to have been born with it, the fuel for her incandescent trajectory from Swansea semi to Hollywood high society. But you needn't be a celebrity, or unconscionably thin or rich, to find your centre and revolve around it (for the record, Dawn French, Beth Ditto and Oprah Winfrey have it too).

Take Rose, a woman I met once at a party some years ago. I've written about her before, but she's well worth revisiting, like an old friend. I was in Lewes, feasting on honeyed madeleines and local wine – and there, among the eclectic mix of guests (a woodsman from a nearby field, a girl with interesting teeth who made organic burgers from her own beef herd, a professional cyclist in yellow Lycra), there was Rose. She was perhaps sixty or thereabouts, with the kind of hair that simply won't behave in public, the colour of steel wool and cut in a nothing-to-speak-of way. She wore no make-up and was broadly as beautiful or as ugly as the next person along. And yet Rose shone. What was it? No Botox. No microdermabrasion. No jumped-up designer clothes. We talked about this and that – a new house, an old joke – while my quizzical eye roamed about to exact the source of her magnetism.

What dawned on me later was that Rose was at one with herself, with her body, her age, her style, her shape. The effect of all this ease was startling. She wore those funky floppy layers that work so well when you're done with the fizzy little explosions of short-order fashion. Rose coupled a charcoal-grey base of skirt and loose shirt with a stunning necklace of silver and amber, heavy with its own history, a necklace with a story to tell, and a capacious shawl of embroidered fabric in claret and tan, which she shrugged closer to her shoulders as the light faded and the temperature dropped in the back yard. The shawl might at one time have draped across a Rajasthani bed, or hung on a wall; it was ethnic, like patchouli, but rare, like gold.

For a seasoned old fashion hack like me, moments of epiphany are, surprisingly, rarer than gold. They were ten a penny when I first started at the catwalk side, wowed by the sheer force of a Gianni Versace show or by Linda Evangelista's legs or by the unutterable perfection of a Dior gown. But through all that, the most potent images of style for me have come from people who understand not the current axioms of fashion, the gossip on the street, the nervous attachment to today's cult handbag or the must-have shoe. They come from people who understand themselves.

This, then, is numinescence – a make-believe word for an unseizable thing. I've encountered it elsewhere too. In my first yoga teacher, for instance, a glorious woman who wore only white and managed to maintain enviable equilibrium and body balance, despite a run-in with breast cancer and subsequent mastectomy. Or my friend Iris, who wears, mostly, wellies and a vast old sweater upon which (I believe) her Golden Retriever once had puppies. She's the kind of woman who finds daisies in her hair, and wears her father's corduroy bags. She's out of synch, but Iris manages the madness by being uncommonly content in her own skin. I envy her in a way I never would a woman in possession of the latest Prada bag (and, believe me, I *love* Prada bags). Or there's the top-rung fashion editor who sailed through the bitch and bustle of the international collections, true always to herself and her style (a series of sober, sophisticated dresses in neutral tones, a wardrobe of perfect shoes), as if she nursed her very own secret, perhaps supplied at a crossroads in return for her soul. I remember watching her out of the corner of my eye as she'd sit at the catwalk side, serene and captivating, while fellow editors squawked and preened, jittery in their Beau Brummell collars, their must-have jackets and monogrammed shoes. While they looked desperate to be someone, anyone else, she looked nonchalantly happy just to be herself.

So how to capture a bit of '*it*' for yourself? By now, you'll have read and absorbed a hundred ways to help you make a start. You'll know that the very act of dieting will inevitably make you feel cruelly dissatisfied with who you are, and that the drip-drip of the diet industry is pure poison, leaving you prone to fast-fix extremism, the snake-oil merchant, the triumph of hopeless optimism over experience.

Losing weight, then, isn't only about the ins and outs of your feeding habits. It's about you and how you feel about yourself. Start with self-acceptance. Start, if you dare, with self-love. It will give you a far more positive and dynamic platform for change, and you won't bore yourself into a hole with the constant drone of self-doubt. As Eleanor Roosevelt had it in one of her oft-quoted epigrams, 'No one can make you feel inferior without your consent.'

'When we are at peace with ourselves,' says psychologist and weight expert Kerry Halliday, 'the body finds its own natural weight. Searching outside ourselves for happiness is one of the reasons we fall prey to the quick fix. Eating problems are often the consequence of a disassociation of self from body. So become physical. Dance. Lighten up. Love yourself again.' You don't have to be a rampant narcissist, but you could give yourself a break. You could stop rewarding yourself with food. You could start today. Couldn't you?

'Losing weight, then, isn't only about the ins and outs of your feeding habits. It's about you and how you feel about yourself.'

NOT A DIET BUT A DO-IT:
HOW TO CAPTURE CONFIDENCE

✴ **Get on your own team**. If you're not on your own cheering section, then why should anyone else be? It's just a basic tenet of good psychiatry. You've got to be positive, yelling 'You can do it!' into the very centre of your soul.

✴ **Know that you are not alone**. A recent survey found that 72 per cent of women rated their looks as 'average' (this is, you'll notice, a statistical impossibility). Interestingly, women who were more satisfied with their own beauty were significantly more likely to think that non-physical factors, including happiness, confidence, dignity, humour, intelligence and wisdom, contribute to making a woman beautiful. Look, no woman on earth loves everything about her body; so find the bits you do. Use this book to help pinpoint them. Cherish them, own them, rely upon them.

✴ **Know what's normal**. Understand that a normal woman, a good woman, can be soft and round. Look at Liv Tyler, a startling beauty who refuses to succumb to Hollywood standards: 'To the rest of the world I am slim,' she says, 'and I like the way I am.'

✴ **Aim for progress, not perfection**. Perfect is excruciatingly dull. It is your fallibility that people will fall for.

✴ **Know who's incredible**. Yep, you are. As Nigella Lawson once quipped, 'Like I say to Charles [Saatchi], I don't ask for much, just 100 per cent adoration all of the time. That's not so unreasonable, is it?' Not to me it's not.

✴ **But do stay alert**. As your body becomes toned and slimmer, sister beware. Success breeds complacency and complacency breeds slackness, which breeds a chirpy little voice inside your head saying that one Custard Cream couldn't possibly hurt. You're right. But three in a row is a recipe for disaster.

Be constant. Staying slim does require will-power; no one is going to do it for you. It's your body, your life, your fudge brownie with hot chocolate sauce, fresh whipped cream and choice of two toppings. Or not.

Be happy. It will keep you in far better shape than being hungry, trust me.

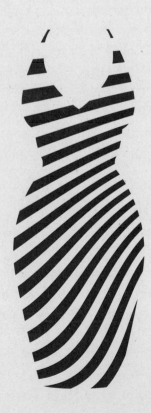

USEFUL WEBSITES

FOOD

fishonline.org for information on sustainable fisheries

mymuesli.com for bespoke muesli

nutritiondata.com for an accurate nutritional breakdown of thousands of food products

UNDERWEAR

axfords.com for corsets

bravissimo.com for 'big-boobed women'

drreyshapewear.com for Dr Rey underwear

everythingunderthedress.com and **usefulchickstuff.co.uk** for Fashion First Aid Boostits, Liftits, Concealits and Tapeits

figleaves.com for Solution Lingerie

rigbyandpeller.com for bra-fitting services

yummietummie.com for T-shirts to trim a tum

FASHION

brownsfashion.com for Preen, and many more brilliant designer labels

duoboots.com and **plusinboots.co.uk** for specialist boot sizes

ilovejeans.com for fabulous jeans in a wide range of sizes

net-a-porter.com for Diane von Furstenburg, Preen, Roland Mouret, Issa

notyourdaughtersjeans.com for Tummy Tuck jeans

miraclesuit.com for the Miracle swimsuit

tightsplease.co.uk for countless versions of the black opaque

HEALTH AND BEAUTY

beautyworkswest.com for Dr Daniel Sister's hormonal health advice

howtolookgood.com for great body shape advice from Caryn Franklin

joannahall.com for the Walk the Weight Off programme and to buy a pedometer

knitty.com for subversive knitters

liftshare.org.uk or **streetcar.co.uk** for car pooling

maccosmetics.com to find your nearest Mac Counter

positivelyslim.com for weight-loss advice from Dr Kerry Halliday

responsibletravel.com, **ecoteer.com**, **originalvolunteer.co.uk**, **peopleandplaces.com**, **yoursafeplanet.co.uk** for volunteer holidays

retouchphoto.co.uk for a picture facelift

stickK.com to put an exercise contract on yourself

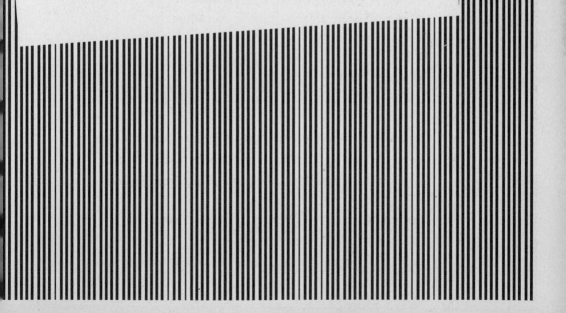

BIBLIOGRAPHY

Bad Food Britain: How a Nation Ruined Its Appetite, by Joanna Blythman (Fourth Estate, 2006).

Cellulite My Arse! by Shonagh Walker (Vermilion, 2003).

Fast Food Nation: What the All-American Meal is Doing to the World, by Eric Schlosser (Penguin, 2002).

I Feel Bad About My Neck, by Nora Ephron (Doubleday, 2007).

In Defense of Food: The Myth of Nutrition and the Pleasures of Eating, by Michael Pollan (Hardcover, 2007).

Mindless Eating: Why We Eat More Than We Think, by Brian Wansink (Bantam-Dell, 2006).

Not on the Label: What Really Goes into the Food on Your Plate, by Felicity Lawrence (Penguin, 2004).

Nudge, by Richard H. Thaler and Cass R. Sunstein (Yale University Press, 2008).

Trans Fat: the Time Bomb in Your Food, by Maggie Stanfield (Souvenir Press, 2008).

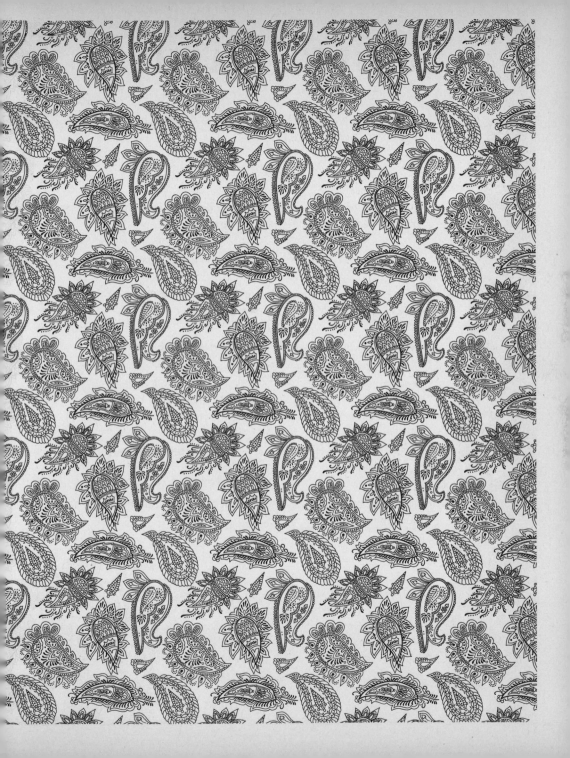

INDEX

NOTES